NURSING HOMES EXPLAINED

Nursing Homes Explained

Delia Marie Franklin

Algora Publishing
New York

Library of Congress Cataloging-in-Publication Data —

Franklin, Delia Marie, 1959-
  Nursing homes explained/ Delia Marie Franklin.
    p. ; cm.
  Includes index.
    ISBN 978-0-87586-966-7 (soft cover : alk. paper) — ISBN 978-0-87586-967-
4 (hard cover : alk. paper) —
    ISBN 978-0-87586-968-1 (ebook)
  I. Title.
    [DNLM: 1. Nursing Homes—organization & administration—United
States. 2. Career Choice—United States. 3. Geriatric Nursing—organization &
administration—United States. 4. Geriatrics—organization & administration—
United States. 5. Long-Term Care—organization & administration—United
States. WX 150 AA1]
    RA997
    362.2'30973—dc23
                         2013008329

Printed in the United States

TABLE OF CONTENTS

INTRODUCTION

Long-term care facilities or nursing homes have been in business for many years in the United States. As the population ages, the quality of healthcare provided in these facilities should be of concern to average individuals within society as well as personnel in the medical profession.

By the year 2030, there will be about 8.1 million people 85 years of age or older in the United States. Longevity is increasing due to healthier lifestyles; better prevention, detection, and treatment of disease processes, and improved education and awareness. As more and more of the population can expect to reach a very advanced age, it is more important for society to have an increased awareness of gerontological nursing, nursing assistant education and training programs, state and federal regulations governing long-term care facilities, the corporate framework guiding the majority of care provided, Medicare and Medicaid funding, state survey processes, customer service, and quality assurance programs in nursing home structure.

The long-term care industry is actually one of the most highly regulated industries in the nation. It has been stated by some that nursing homes are actually regulated more strictly than nuclear power plants. Federal regulatory statutes set guidelines to be followed in the nursing home industry; but corporations, private sector owners, and state surveyors need to insure regulations are being implemented and followed in nursing home facilities throughout the nation.

Gerontological nursing is a very rewarding career choice for personnel in the medical profession. For individuals to be able to increase their knowledge base about the aging process, death and dying, disease processes, and regulatory initiatives to improve the quality of life and death for the elderly in our nation is a very positive attribute to society. The long-term care industry, unfortunately a lot of times is not presented in a very positive light to society, creating false perceptions in individual's psychology about this industry. There are positive and negative qualities about nursing home facilities, but there are positive and negative qualities about every aspect of the healthcare continuum within the medical profession.

Improving social awareness of positive attributes accredited to the long-term industry, and identifying some of the challenges in this industry will generate an interdisciplinary approach in society and medical profession; hopefully increasing levels of quality of care services provided to the elderly in our nation. Elderly clients and their family systems deserve to have high level quality of services provided to them when placed in a nursing home setting. Family members deserve to have peace of mind about the care and services provided to their loved one's while residing in a long-term care facility. By increasing social awareness and educational levels about this process in life, as concerned individuals we can expand on and improve our care to the elderly within society.

Educational processes are going to be presented in a way that I hope will be both entertaining and educational to the reader. Through the utilization of humor, issues in life can sometimes be handled more positively and effectively when attempting to improve systems. I have found that humor utilized appropriately in the long-term care industry is a very positive force to implement with clients; it improves their day and contributes to the quality of their life.

Clients also being of keen wit in a lot of cases will utilize humor with staff improving morale and well-being for all individuals in a facility. The amount of workload and level of quality of care encompassing gerontological clients can be demanding and stressful for both staff and clients in long-term care facilities, contributing to burnout and high staff turnover rates in the industry. If a small factor like humor can help improve the psychological well-being for human beings on all levels in a facility, then why not utilize the tool when appropriate to improve quality of life. Humor will be utilized throughout the material presented and hopefully it will be viewed from a positive perspective to assist the elderly population in our nation.

Chapter One. Corporations

It is estimated that only 20–30% of the geriatric population in the world are admitted to nursing home facilities. The majority of elderly individuals remain in their residential environments and never experience a nursing home setting. The age range of the population in long-term care facilities is generally about 80–100. Each gerontological client is as individualized as the institutions they reside in, generating a uniquely interesting living and working environment within the medical profession.

While assisting the geriatric population, society must understand that the human brain does not age with the body and this phenomena explains why some elderly individuals at the age of 86 or above will sky dive, climb mountains, perform aerobic exercises, water and snow ski, Para glide etc.....The majority of the geriatric population has psychologically conceptualized their own mortality and has matured to the emotional and psychological level of acceptance of death as an inevitable part of life.

Let's explore the long-term care industry by first examining corporations and corporate structure. The LTC (long-term care) industry has both corporate owned and private sector facilities in the United States. Corporate owned facilities have many positive attributes accredited to them in the nation, but also have some challenges within nursing home structure. Senior level management gears middle management strategies with decision-making processes in corporate owned facilities. In private sector nursing home facilities, middle management has more autonomy with decision-making processes in regards to business decisions, but they do not have corporate resources for improvement with quality of education and healthcare. Some major long-term care corporations in the United States are Five Star Senior Living, Vetter Health Services, Inc., Golden Living Centers, Evangelical Lutheran Good Samaritan Society, Deseret Health Group, and Sava Senior Care.

Corporate Structure

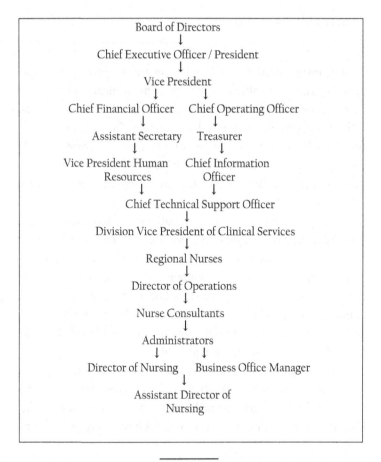

In the long-term care industry a chain of command is followed when addressing concerns at a senior management level. The Chief Executive Officer is generally contacted by the Director of Operations when issues present themselves that require upper level management assistance. The diagram on the facing page depicts senior chain-of-command levels in the corporate long-term care industry.

Chief Executive Officers

In the long-term care industry a CEO (chief executive officer) is one of the highest-ranking officers in charge of total management within the corporate structure. An individual in this position reports directly to the Board of Directors in the long-term care industry. A CEO must possess a balance between internal and external initiatives to build a sustainable corporation that aligns with their strategic vision. Core duties of this position include facilitating business strategies outside of the corporation, while guiding employees and executive officers towards a central objective for a specific long-term care corporation. A CEO should coordinate external initiatives for a corporation at a high level of performance.

It is stated by some individuals that to be a strong executive "one cannot act in business differently from how an individual acts in family life or society." Meaning an individual's actions must follow their words at all times to be successful in this type of position.

A Chief Executive Officer in the long-term care industry must possess at least a Bachelor's degree, but a graduate degree in business, health care administration, social sciences, or a health care profession is the preferred educational level for an individual in this position within nursing home structure. Proven abilities to successfully resolve conflicts, and to exercise independent and effective judgment on an ongoing basis, are needed skills for a Chief Executive Officer. Responsibilities and duties for a Chief Executive Officer in the long-term care industry may include:

- Providing administration and supervision of leadership, operation, and management of the corporation with guidance from the board of directors.
- Assisting with the selection, hiring and training of new board members.
- Collaborating with the board for preparation and conduction of board meetings.
- Examining policies and bylaws on a regular basis to ensure corporate compliance with such laws and standards.
- Maintaining budgetary review records and presenting information to the board of directors.
- Formulating corporate strategic direction with short and long term goals developed and implemented with board input and assistance.
- Supervising overall operations to insure in accordance with legal, regulatory, licensure, and accreditation standards.
- Maintaining effective marketing and advertising strategies that have measurable goals.
- Ensuring an executive assistant is maintained on staff to assume leadership in the absence of the chief executive officer.
- Demonstrating support and maintaining fund raising operations.
- Effectively participating in team building through mentoring, educating, and inspiring employees at all levels in the corporate setting.

Subordinate executives for a Chief Executive Officer in the long-term care industry typically include a —

CFO (chief financial officer)
COO (chief operating officer)
CTO (chief technical officer)
CIO (chief information officer)
Vice President of Human Resources

Director of Operations

Corporations in the long-term care industry utilize employees in the position of (DO) Director of Operations and this usually consists of one individual in each state. This position entails someone who directs, administers, and coordinates activities of the corporation in support of policies, goals, and objectives established by the CEO and Board of Directors by performing duties personally or through administrative personnel. An individual in this position also assists the Chief Executive Officer with development of corporate policies, procedures and goals that entail operations, personnel, financial performance, and growth. Major responsibilities surrounding a director's position guide and regulate management in the development, promotion, and financial aspects of a corporation's delivered services.

A Director of Operations in the long-term care industry should possess a focus in areas that establish preparation of short-term and long-range plans, including budgets based on broad organizational and growth objectives in the areas of —

> *Support Services*
> *Business Development*
> *Program Planning/Development*
> *Information Technology*
> *Human Resources*
> *Managed Care Operations*
> *Health Care Policy*

The Director of Operations implements programs and oversees facility directors; ensuring they meet corporate policies, goals, and objectives in the nursing home setting. Developing procedures, installing procedures, and implementing controls to promote communication and adequate information flow within a corporation are an essential component of this position. A Director of Operations establishes operating policies and evaluates the overall results of operations regularly and systematically; reporting these results to the Chief Executive Officer within organizational long-term care structure.

An ability to delegate portions of activities, responsibilities, and authorities as necessary and desirable to organizational staff, and to general managers/directors is a needed expertise for an individual at this level of corporate structure. In conjunction with the Chief Executive Officer, a Director of Operations ensures that all organization activities and operations are carried out in compliance with local, state, and federal regulations and bylaws governing business operations within long-term care structure. A Director of Operations in the long-term care industry must possess knowledge and expertise in the areas of —

Clinical Operations/Licensing   Program Development
Budget Preparation   Grant Management
Managed Care Operations   Finance
Health Policy   Business Development
Fund Raising
Maintaining private, state, federal and local relationships to advance initiatives for a corporation.

An individual in the position of Director of Operations needs to be able to assess, evaluate, and implement strategies in facilities that improve client care, while balancing monetary aspects of the corporation for a state.

Some individuals in the Director of Operations position follow examples set by a CEO and Board of Directors, and some develop egos, with a perception that they can set their own path for a corporation. It does create dysfunction in a corporate setting when senior level management are not on the same page, or in some cases, not even in the same book with the mission and vision set by a CEO and Board for a business. Group psychology in senior level management needs to be congruent; facilitating an environment that assists middle management in the facilities on a daily basis. Similar psychological processes will work to accomplish the goal of obtaining a mission and vision for a corporation through improvement of quality of care for clients in the multidisciplinary approach with care delivery systems.

Some individuals employed in the Director of Operation position participate in political game playing within corporate structure and in long-term care facilities to achieve a potential gain for them self in the medical profession. This type of leader is not what this industry needs; a focus for the long-term care industry should always be on improvement of quality of care delivery systems for the client, and meeting a mission and vision of a CEO and Board of Directors in a corporation. When a Director of Operations ventures off on their own path within a corporate setting it usually does not end with positive results for the individual or for the facilities that they are responsible for managing, which unfortunately then trickles down to the client.

Gerontological patients deserve to have leaders in senior level management positions that are focused on them and their needs in the long-term care industry structure. Chief Executive Officers a lot of times inherit individuals in a Director of Operations position from a previous corporate structure; with this in mind, a CEO needs to evaluate the psychology of individuals in a Director of Operations position, and establish whether the DO's vision really is what the CEO wants to support as a goal for accomplishment in their corporate setting.

Nurse Consultants

Corporate owned long-term care facilities maintain nurse consultants and regional nurses on staff that they utilize to improve and maintain quality of care delivery services in their facilities. Private sector facilities do not have these nurse positions to utilize on staff, but there are some organizations within society that these facilities can utilize to hire a nurse consultant for improvement of care delivery systems. Hired consultants will assess nursing homes systems and make recommendations for improvement of quality of care in nursing home structure.

Regional nurses or nurse consultants provide consultation and technical assistance to medical professionals and the public on all aspects of a nursing specialty, such as gerontology. Consultant nurses will —

> *Provide advice and guidance.*
> *Utilize established protocols.*
> *Develop and deliver training in a specific nursing specialty.*
> *Collect and analyze data for use in program development and evaluation.*
> *Audit healthcare delivery systems for adherence to established nursing standards.*

A nurse consultant in the long-term care industry should be fully proficient and knowledgeable about all aspects of gerontological clients, geriatric nursing, state and federal mandated regulations, nursing home management, corporate structure and management, state survey processes, and systems required to maintain and sustain a high quality level of care for clients in the nursing home environment. The nurse consultant position is distinguished from other nursing series, as it focuses on consultation and technical assistance to healthcare professionals and managers rather than on the delivery or supervision of direct care nursing services. Examples of duties for a gerontological nurse consultant position may include:

- Providing clinical nursing and program consultation, including onsite technical assistance to healthcare professionals following established protocols and practices in long-term care facilities.

- Assisting health care managers by providing information and formulating recommendations affecting changes to policies and procedures, protocols, and practices at corporate and facility levels.

- Identifying and anticipating needs and potential problem areas in the nursing home environment.

- Advising operational health managers and administrators on strategies in the delivery of nursing services on all levels in the long-term care arena.

- Conducting audits of nursing practice in the facilities allotted for their region.

- Implementing quality assurance practices at corporate and facility levels.

- Developing and delivering staff training.

- Potentially assisting in the development and practice of research studies in a specific nursing practice such as gerontology.

Specialty nurse consultants in the long-term care industry must possess knowledge, skills, and abilities surrounding gerontological nursing. A nurse in this position needs to have a thorough knowledge of current nursing principles, practices, and procedures; plus understand current philosophies and methodology of nursing practice, health promotion, and disease prevention in the nursing home environment. Considerable knowledge of healthcare, healthcare delivery systems, and governmental requirements related to gerontological nursing is a necessity for a long-term care nurse consultant. A gerontological nurse consultant position also requires an individual to possess understanding of research principles and methodology; principles and methods of consultation; role responsibility, and interrelationships of various health disciplines and health agencies within society. An ability to conduct investigations and assessments, provide justification to support findings, participate in research, and assisting with implementing protocols are requirements for a nurse consultant in long-term care structure. The gerontological nurse must articulate well and communicate effectively in both oral and written forms. A nurse consultant position requires the individual to possess an ability to analyze situations accurately and take effective action, plus nurses must be flexible and innovative in their approaches to the resolution of problems within the industry.

A major short and long term goal for nurse consultants within the long-term care industry is the improvement and maintenance of state survey processes. Annual surveys that depict positive outcomes demonstrate a high quality level of care; improving reputations of facilities, increasing clientele admission census, and generating maintenance of monetary revenue. Maintenance of monetary revenue generates financial stability for corporations in the long-term care industry.

An individual employed as a gerontological nurse consultant should have experience in a DNS (Director Nursing Services) position with demonstrated positive survey results in the long-term care setting. It is difficult for a nurse to establish systems in an environment that they do not intellectually know or understand. Just being a nurse (whether BSN or MSN) will not provide an individual with the knowledge of experience (theory is not applicable in all situations.) Experience provides nurses with a knowledge base of which systems and techniques work or do not work to improve levels of care delivery systems in a nursing home environment.

Consultants are required to come into their designated facilities on a monthly basis to evaluate care standards, policies and procedures, environmental standards, medical records, rehabilitative services, minimum data set documentation, etc... Gerontological nurse consultants do have a set psychology with improvement of quality of care delivery systems, but a problem can arise when the individual does not possess knowledge base of what systems to integrate in nursing home structure to accomplish the goal of improvement of care in a facility. Or, if the consultant has a Director of Nursing in a building that is not willing to put in the hours to accomplish the corporation's goals. Gerontological nurse consultants require middle management support to assist in accomplishing their goals encompassing quality of care delivery systems in a nursing home environment.

Regional nurses are corporate management nurse positions that usually require a master's degree in nursing. Nurses in these positions oversee nurse consultants, and usually have a multi-state region that they manage. Regional nurses write policies and procedures that are incorporated into nursing home facilities that are corporate-owned and operated. A regional nurse must possess an expert knowledge base of state and federal rules and regulations that govern practices in long-term care facilities. A minor educational degree in business structure is beneficial with a Regional Nurse Position.

> The Regional Nurse Director will assess, develop, evaluate and implement clinical service operations in an assigned geographic area.

Gerontological Regional Nurses also assist with ensuring compliance with federal and state regulations, company standards of care, and corporate operational practices. Trends of best practices and potential risks will be identified in nursing home structure during regional nurse assessment processes, and regional nurses incorporate their findings into process improvements within the industry. Regional nurses will also assist in nursing department budget planning for long-term care facilities. Participation in quality improvement systems in the areas of nursing, dietary, activities, social services, and clinical information management are included in a Gerontological Regional Nurse job performance within the long-term care industry.

The Vice President of Clinical Services manages corporate nurses at a regional or consultant level in long-term care facilities. Areas of this position encompass overseeing quality clinical operations and services to clients within a specific division. Systems in nursing, dietary, social services, rehabilitation, activities, medical records, and administration are assessed and quality improvement processes implemented to sustain and maintain quality of care. A VP of Clinical Services maintains compliance with federal and state regulations, OBRA requirements, and company policies and procedures within divisional facilities.

Mission Statements

Mission statements are a commonly utilized strategy in corporate-owned long-term care facilities, and they depict a formal short written summary of the purpose of a company or corporation. A mission statement should —

> *Act as a guideline for the actions of a corporation*
> *Explain the overall goal surrounding corporate structure*
> *Give a sense of direction for senior management*
> *Assist in decision-making processes for all employees*

When a corporation's mission statement is written it should be broad enough to allow for creative growth, distinguish a corporation from all others in an industry, serve as a framework to evaluate current activities, and be stated clearly so it is understood by all who read it in society.

Mission statements provide a "framework" in which strategies are formulated. (The word "mission" dates from 1598, originally from the Jesuits—"missio" is Latin for the "act of sending [abroad]."

A mission statement should contain—

- An explanation for the reason for the existence of a corporation. (mission)
- A depiction of some future state for the corporation. (vision)
- A representation of the key values within a corporation.
- The major goals envisioned for a corporation.

While visionary goals are selected, core values and purpose of a corporation should be discovered during the goal selection process.

Values and purpose should be set in a corporation's structure at the initiation of its existence; a mission statement just describes them, making customers more likely to believe a corporation's mission.

Customers, including family members and patients need to evaluate a corporate owned facilities mission statement and determine if staff in a facility actually follows the vision and mission incorporated by a company. Mission statements do attempt to set a certain psychology for individuals in the long-term care industry, yet middle management in a facility may differ in mental processes. Middle management teams at times can dictate a different philosophy of thinking than a corporation, which may lead to deterrence in obtaining corporate goals.

Corporate-Owned and Private Sector

Knowledge base about both types of facilities, corporate owned and private sector, does not allow individuals in the health care profession the opportunity to provide recommendations to anyone on which to choose for their beloved family member. Each family system needs to evaluate the loved one's needs and the family's needs, then make a decision based on what will work best for the family's situation. Family systems will need to evaluate —

Location	*Type of Facility*
Patients Medical Condition	*Monetary Resources*
Disease Processes	*Services Provided*
State Survey	*Inspection Records*
General Disposition and Attitudes of Staff	

Elderly clients do rely on their family members to research nursing home placement and derive a decision that will work best for all involved in the long-term care admission process. The transition of loss and change can be difficult for clients prior, during and after admission. All individuals involved with transition processes should display extra kindness and compassion towards clients until they adjust to their new living arrangement.

We will mention only a few of the corporations in operation within the nation to give you a general idea of their philosophies and missions within this industry.

Five Star Senior Living

Five Star Senior Living, which emerged during a financial process concerning Integrated Health Services; owns over 200 facilities in the United States and is a financially stable corporation. Corporate headquarters are in Newton, Massachusetts. Clients have relayed some very positive experiences while residing in their facilities. In the year 2011, the President and CEO (chief executive officer) position belonged to Bruce J. Mackey, Jr. CPA (certified public accountant.) Senior level management consists of several individuals and I will list a couple: Paul V. Hoagland, CPA Treasurer, Chief Financial Officer; Rosemary Esposito RN, Senior Vice President, and Chief Operating Officer; Janet E. Mercier, Vice President and Director of Human Resources; Travis K. Smith, Attorney, Vice President and General Counsel to Secretary. Divisional Vice Presidents include: Jerry Andreatos, Eastern Division; Scott Herzig, Western Division; Steve Johnson, Midwest Division; and Kerri Nielsen, Rehabilitation, Hospitals and Pharmacy Division. Denise Kelly is the Vice President of Rehabilitation and Wellness. The corporation's upper management team consists of some well-educated, highly qualified individuals that instill systems for producing high-level quality customer service. Five individuals are included in the Board of Directors for this corporation.

The corporation's mission statement and values consists of five stars that they follow surrounding services rendered.

> 1 – We mind the business; build upon a solid financial base, carefully manage assets and translate bottom line results into even better resident care.
>
> 2 – We are accountable, work to be our best and go the extra mile.
>
> 3 – We listen and then act decisively, we have a bias for action.
>
> 4 – We put people first, we help each other
>
> 5 – We act with integrity, we are trusting and trust worthy.

All long-term care facilities are rated through the United States Health and Human Services Department (Nursing Homes Compare) in four areas including an overall rating, health inspections, nursing home staffing and quality measures. Several facilities owned by this corporation rank four to five stars in all four areas of assessment by the Health and Human Services Department.

The corporation itself portrays a positive effort to improve the quality of care for the gerontological client and puts systems into place to obtain and maintain that goal. The first CEO Everett Benton is a man with integrity, wisdom, morals, and values and he implemented those qualities into the corporation's framework. Beliefs, attitudes, values and practices of senior level management will set the practice and tone of an entire corporation; group psychology does demonstrate that members of a team will follow examples set by leaders in nursing home structure.

Family members need to evaluate the leaders in a facility and corporation; subordinate employees will display the leaders in middle or senior level management positions behaviors and practices in a long-term care environment. If complaints are not handled from a positive perspective to improve quality of care, but role reversal is utilized to blame family members or a patient for perceived problems, then family members need to reevaluate the situation of client placement. Elderly clients have enough problems dealing with their bodily changes and disease processes; they do not need employee behaviors to add to their repertoire of problems. Leaders that demonstrate healthy relationship interactions with positive problem solving skills are present in the Five Star Senior Living corporate structure.

Golden Living Centers

Golden Living Centers formerly known as Beverly Healthcare has its corporate headquarters in Fort Smith, Arkansas and owns approximately 300 facilities in 21 states. This corporation has had some challenges in the industry. Financial stability does exist at this current time. Golden Innovations a sub-branch of Golden Living, includes Aseracare (hospice services) and Aegis Therapy. Neil Kurtz, MD occupied the President and CEO position of Golden Living in 2011. James Avery, MD is the Senior Vice President and Chief

Medical Officer of Golden Living. Cindy Susienka is the Corporations President and CEO of Golden Innovations and Larry Deans is the President of Golden Living Centers.

A mission statement of "Experience the Golden Difference" redefining healthcare for seniors depicts a psychological conception of high quality care and improving quality of services.

The company has a code of conduct and business ethics that serves as guidance to employees; it sets forth legal and ethical standards for the corporation's employees.

The corporation definitively puts systems into action to improve quality of care for clients, as demonstrated when they hired two state nurses: one a federal regulatory nurse for a specific state and one a regulatory MDS (minimum data set) nurse coordinator for a specific state. The state nurses implemented systems within the corporate structure to meet regulatory standards within their facilities, thus improving quality of care for clients in the nursing home environment. Conversations with clients in the facilities during their visits to assess care levels, patient satisfaction with staffing, and facility healthcare delivery systems showed that the clients perceived that the state nurses set a standard for the corporation.

It is impressive when senior level management displays an interest in the quality of care clients are being provided and a concern with satisfaction in their living arrangements.

Senior level management in this corporation also includes: Andrea Clark, Senior Vice President of Clinical services; John O'Conner, Vice President Clinical Services Aegis Rehab; Liz Grima, Senior Vice President Human Resource Services; and John Derr, Chief Technology Strategic Officer. United States Health and Human Services (Nursing Homes Compare) star ratings range from one to four stars in most of their facilities in relation to all four areas of evaluation.

Evangelical Lutheran Good Samaritan Society

Evangelical Lutheran Good Samaritan Society encompasses facilities in 230 locations in the United States. Corporate headquarters are located in Sioux Falls, South Dakota. The corporation was founded in 1922 by Reverend August Hoeger in Arthur, North Dakota. The corporation's vision is to create an environment where people are loved, valued and at peace based on four core principles—

Compassion	*Vocation*
Hospitality	*Service*

A mission statement depicts the corporation's psychology:

"In Christ's Love Everyone Is Someone" reminds all present to share God's love in word and deed by providing shelter and supportive services to older persons and others in need in the nation.

In 2011, the president and CEO of this corporation was David J. Harezdovsky. Senior level management consists of 11 positions including: Cynthia L. Mosenburg, Executive Vice President for Regional Operations; Raye Nae Nylanders, Executive Vice President for Financial Services; Neal Eddy, Vice President learning and strategic integration; Thomas J. Kapusta, Vice President Legal Audit and Compliance Services; William Kubat, Vice President for resident, community, and quality services; Dean Mertz, Vice President Human Resources; and Rustan Williams, Vice President Information Services and Technology.

The corporation has a foundation and Charles Hiatt is the foundation's Executive Director. Corporate description of their foundation consists of an entity that gathers, grows and provides the channels through which gifts and grants flow to support and improve the quality of life for those in our care. Board of Directors consists of 16 individuals; John C. Penn is the Chairman of the Board and resides in Hopkins, MN. United States Health and Human Services (Nursing Homes Compare) star ratings consist of one to five stars in all four areas of assessment in most of the corporations facilities.

Sava Senior Care

Sava Senior Care merged with Mariner Health Care in 2004. The corporation owns 190 facilities in the nation with corporate headquarters in Atlanta, Georgia. A mission statement "Focus on people, our residents, their lives, and their families" encompasses the philosophy of this organization. In 2011, some of the executives that managed the corporation included: Tony Ololsby, President and CEO; Thomas Simons, Chief Financial Officer; Leonard Grunstein, Chairman; Robert Lyle, Vice President and Controller; Mark Janek, Director Information Technology; and Peter Lougee, President, Western Division. United States Health and Human Services (Nursing Homes Compare) star rating consists of one to three stars in all four areas within their facilities.

Vetter Health Services

Vetter Health Services, Inc. owns 33 facilities in 5 states. Corporate headquarters is in Elkhorn, NE. Jack Vetter is the founder, CEO, and Chairman of the corporation. Mr. Vetter purchased his first nursing home in 1975 in Fairbury, NE.

> The corporation's mission statement is "Dignity in Life" the Vetter way.

A Vetter Vision guides psychological processes of the corporation in areas surrounding —

Quality of Life	*Quality of Care*
Excellent Teams	*Outstanding Facilities*
Quality Reputation	*Stewardship*

Their values include —

> Serving: *Focus on exceeding people's expectations*
> Integrity: *Act with honesty, fairness, and compassion*
> Teamwork: *Relationships built on trust and respect*
> Excellence: *Continually pursues opportunities to improve*

Senior level management in 2011 included Glen Van Ekeran, President; Patrick Fairbanks, Chief Operations Officer; Joan Schelm, Chief Financial Officer; and Mitchell Elliott, Chief Developmental Officer. The Vetter foundation was founded in 1992 and is explained as a system to provide support for worldwide mission work. United States Health and Human Services (Nursing Homes Compare) star ratings range from one to five regarding all four areas of assessment in their facilities.

Deseret Health Group

Deseret Health Group was founded in 2006 by Jon H. Robertson within the state of Utah. Deseret is a term utilized in the Mormon Bible that means "honeybee." The corporation displays a philosophy surrounding, "A passion for life. A place for caring."

> "Our family philosophy ensures your loved ones are respected and cared for by the most professional staff with regard to their health, individuality, and dignity."

The corporation owns 24 nursing homes located in Nebraska, Utah, Kansas, and Minnesota. Encompassing a vision of displaying healthcare with a heart in the Midwest region of the United States; Deseret is moving forward and progressing in growth within the long-term care industry. The executive team consists of Chief Executive Officer, Garett Robertson; Chief Operating Officer, Scott D. Stringham; Chief Financial Officer, Lars Elliott; and Regional VP of Operations, Clayton South.

The facilities owned by this corporation demonstrate one to five stars in the Health and Human Services rating systems within the nation.

Private Sector Facilities

Private owned facilities evaluated for the discussion process appeared to rank higher in the United States, Health and Human Services (Nursing Homes Compare) star rating process. Most facilities rated between, three to five in the four areas of assessment by the government. This may demonstrate that the overall rating, health inspections, nursing home staffing, and quality measures are in a higher-ranking quality for private owned facilities. Private owned nursing homes do not have corporations to dictate their staffing ratios, which may translate into a perceived better quality of care for the patient in some circumstances.

Observers of nursing home structure will tell you that this perception is not always reality based. These institutions do not have corporate resources for implementation of systems to monitor and improve quality assurance processes, including policies and procedures utilized in their facilities. Quality improvement of systems in these facilities will require nurses that are trained by corporations to go into their facilities; evaluate systems in place and instill changes to improve the level of healthcare in their nursing homes. Even though the staff to patient ratio may be above corporate owned facilities, if middle management does not have the education and knowledge base entailing how to improve the level of systems implemented in their facilities, longevity with quality of care will not be a maintained entity for these facilities.

Some private sector nursing homes state their mission in the long-term care industry and some do not have mission statements formulated for their business structure.

One facility relayed their mission as emphasizing ethical, respectful, and compassionate nursing care by meeting the needs and exceeding the expectations of the residents, their families, and the communities we serve, and establishing ourselves as the premier healthcare employer for professional, progressive employees.

Another private sector facility operated under Rural Health Development Consulting and Management stated their mission as:

"The cornerstone of all success is the quality of our people and all clients....a series of relationships that set the standards for our industry."

Focus

Corporations in the long-term care industry are a very positive entity to initiate high quality healthcare delivery systems to the gerontological client. Individuals in these positions do possess a mission and vision to provide all gerontological patients with high quality care in the nation. Senior level management personnel do implement mission statements, business structure systems, policies and procedures, and healthcare delivery systems that foster high quality level care to all clients within a corporation setting. Knowing that individuals in these positions do not just sit in their offices at corporate headquarters, but actually go into facilities in the nation demonstrates that they do care about the perceptions of their corporation and nursing home environment within society.

Society needs to be aware that the majority of senior level management staff in corporate-owned facilities work very hard to achieve and sustain high level care delivery systems to manage facilities owned by a corporation in the nation.

Executives ask about care delivery systems and whether clients are satisfied with the nursing services provided; this is a definitive example of their involvement level.

An individual with this much power in a business, visiting clients to inquire about the services provided and the clients perceived satisfaction with services rendered in a nursing home, demonstrates that senior level management in the long-term care corporate structure do perform their jobs at a high standard in the industry. Negative perceptions of corporations and nursing homes in general are formulated within society because of a relatively minor number of negative situations that do transpire in long-term care facilities.

Public awareness is made national when negative situations occur in a facility, yet all of the positive high level structure and systems that transpire on a daily basis is never acknowledged within the media, creating a perception that is not reality based in most long-term care facilities. Hopefully, the remainder of our exploration will assist the nation to view the long-term care industry as a positive force in the health care continuum that works to assist our elderly to receive the best quality of care that can be provided for them in our nursing homes within the nation

CHAPTER TWO. MIDDLE MANAGEMENT

Middle management positions are a rewarding and sometimes challenging employment opportunity in the long-term care industry. Administrators and Director of Nurses occupy middle management positions in long-term care facilities within the nation. The word management itself comes from two sources —

> Old French "menagement – the art of conducting and directing"
> Latin "manu agere – to lead by hand"

Thus, management can be thought of as the process of leading and directing a business through the skillful deployment of resources, including actions measuring quality and quantity in a timely fashion, and adjusting plans as needed to obtain an intended goal.

Positions encompassing middle management skills in the medical profession can generate more stress than other positions in the geriatric healthcare continuum. Individuals employed in middle management positions are pressed from two sides, senior level management and line staff. Middle management employees are the individuals that incorporate systems to maintain compliance with regulatory guidelines in long-term care facilities, and the requirement for strategic thinking processes is a necessity to motivate line staff with implementation of improvement systems. Staff burnout, which we will discuss at a later time, is a factor to take into consideration with any changes incorporated in a long-term care facility in the industry.

History of Corporate Management

A historical viewpoint of management can be traced back to ancient Egyptian pyramid builders; management as a resource for conducting work projects has existed for centuries in the world. Management as a business discipline emerged in the 19th century due to economic declines in the nation. Theories on management began evolving in the 20th century around the year 1920. In the 1940s, operations research initiated also known as "management science" which took a scientific avenue to management problems in the areas of logistics and operations. Progressing towards the end of the 20th century management moved into specific branches such as human resource management, operations management, strategic management, marketing management, financial management, and information technology management. In the 21st century, management progressed into a thought process of various areas or regions that require the skillful deployment of management including —

Change	*Communication*
Cost	*Crisis*
Customer Service	*Facilities*
Knowledge	*Marketing*
Programs	*Systems*
Risk	*Time*
Quality	*Perceptions*

The middle management position is a key tool surrounding communication processes between line staff and senior level management in corporate structure. Managers in middle management positions are representatives of a corporation; reflecting a company's standards and values to other managers, line staff and customers in a business setting. Middle managers are the individuals that bear the largest responsibility for developing and maintaining quality management in a long-term care facility, and are considered the layer of management in an organization whose primary job responsibility is to monitor activities of subordinates and report their observations, evaluations and strategic management outcomes to senior level management personnel within the long-term care corporate setting.

Middle managers are the individuals that implement systems, policies and procedures within long-term care structure that are developed in senior level management corporate initiatives to improve conduction of business in a nursing home. Quality of management strategies utilized by middle managers in the long-term care industry has a strong influence in the areas of customer satisfaction, employee morale, and the success of a specific nursing home or corporation within society.

Administrators

Administrators are a needed equipoise in the long-term care spectrum. An administrator directs the operations of a long-term care facility on a 24-hour a day basis and should maintain a professional high quality level of operation seven days per week. High quality level patient care and services rendered are required to meet the satisfaction of clients, family members and physicians; minimizing deficiencies, complaints and lawsuits within the long-term care industry.

In corporate owned facilities the administrator implements policies and procedures (in private owned facilities writing the policies and procedure may be a task requirement) to comply with federal, state, local and corporation bylaws and regulations to meet licensure certification standards for a nursing home. Administrators in the long-term care arena are responsible for facility management, profitability, operations and directions within their facility. Management regions can include —

Census	Net Operating Income
Patient Care	Survey Compliance
Employee Relations	Accounts Receivable and Collections
Positive Return on Investment	

A long-term care nursing home administrator develops, implements, and maintains a facility budget to comply with corporate policy and procedures or county/corporate board directives in the long-term care industry. An individual in this position evaluates occupancy rates; staff to patient ratios; and private pay, Medicare, Medicaid payment resources to maintain revenue; sustaining financial operational functions of a facility. Administrators will confer with Medical Directors and nurse consultants to ensure compliance with regulatory guidelines and to maintain a high level quality of care in a facility. Participating in various committee meetings to implement, maintain and sustain quality assurance measures is a requirement with an administrator job description. Hiring personnel, analyzing job performance through evaluation processes, plus directing and terminating department heads are a required duty in an administrator position in nursing home structure.

Some administrators will perform survey processes with employees and clients to determine satisfaction with a Director of Nursing in some long-term care facilities.

It is an interesting process to examine different perceptions of individuals with middle management positions. Within the long-term care industry there can be variances in psychological perceptions regarding middle management staff, usually the majority of comments are positive in survey processes, but some employees can sustain completely negative perceptions of a nurse and view everything a nurse does as wrong or incorrect for a facility. Negative thinking processes can deter management effectiveness in a long-term care facility; group negativity will decrease goal obtainment with management strategies within this industry.

An administrator serves as a primary liaison for patients, families, staff, and the general public in the nursing home setting. Problem solving skills are a necessity in an administrator position to sustain group cohesiveness in a facility. Essential functions may include but are not limited to —

Supervisory Responsibilities	*Business Planning*
Accounts Receivable	*Census/Mix Management*
Net Operating Income	*Labor and Workforce Planning*
Reimbursement	*Patient Trust Accounts*
Consumer Satisfaction	*Performance Evaluating*
Risk Management	*Environmental Improvements*
Budget Strategies	*Compliance*

Minimum requirements for a nursing home administrator are that they be licensed in the state of practice as an administrator. There are courses at community colleges to prepare an individual to test for a nursing home administrator license. Some corporations require their administrators to have a Bachelor's degree in business administration to be employed in an Administrator's position within their facilities. Some administrators do display a sense of humor with their job performance as the following scenario depicts.

During a state survey process the nursing home prepared and held a celebration party while the state survey inspection was being conducted in the facility. The party encompassed a magician performing magic acts for clients and family members. During the administrators introductions at the initiation of the party the state surveyors were walking past the party room and the administrator invited them into the room to introduce them to the individuals present for the celebration.

> While introducing both surveyors the administrator stated, "And for an encore presentation, our magician is going to make the surveyors disappear."

> One of the surveyors rang back, "Not as fast as you think."

Staff and clients both laughed at the scenario and it lightened the mood for the party process. A sense of humor in the long-term care arena when applied properly is a positive asset to assist with staff morale and client satisfaction within the nursing home environment.

Staff appreciation and improvement committees are formulated in some facilities and meet on a monthly basis to evaluate, structure and implement strategies for staff morale, retention, and increased quality care processes to assist in positive approaches with staffing management in specific nursing homes. Motivational gifts for staff can be purchased by middle management to demonstrate appreciation for desired work performance such as Bath and Body Works perfumes and soaps, nursing tee-shirts, corporate sweatshirts, nurse aide tote bags, and various gift certificates to name a few; assisting in inter-employee relationship development within nursing home facilities.

Elaborating on different stories, experiences and strategies experienced or encountered in long-term care facilities will hopefully assist the public to view this industry from a new or different, and appreciated perspective within the healthcare continuum. William's case displays the required need for compassion surrounding employee psychology in the industry.

William's story

William was diagnosed with schizophrenia and mental retardation. He resided in a long-term care facility from the age of 36 until his death. William was a favorite client of many employees in the nursing home he lived in during his life.

William possessed a stuffed ball that had a voice activated mechanism in it that when thrown and hit against an object would elicit the sound Ha! Ha! Ha! While residing in the long-term care facility, a nurse decided to toss the ball to William, attempting to initiate a game of catch with the patient. William's mental retardation made him unable to understand the nurse's actions, and he was frightened. William started trembling and shaking due to confusion over the nurse's behavior.

The nurse called in a second nurse to demonstrate to William how to play toss with a ball.

The simple dynamic of playing toss initiated a different relationship between the nurse and William, changing interactions in the nursing home setting. Every time the nurse walked out of her office, William would toss the ball to her, verbalizing Ha! Ha! Ha! The nurse would toss the ball back and William would catch it, waiting until she arrived in his presence again to continue the game.

Not knowing what mannerisms or social behaviors are appropriate or inappropriate; William would go into the nursing office, sit down and watch the nurses work for extended periods of time, and would laugh at them at times.

William, even with his disabilities, was able to develop a level of trust with some staff members, due to the client–staff relationship development through a simple game of "toss the ball." Staff were able to shave, cut nails, trim his mustache, and catheterize William without any fear or discontent with the hygiene and medical procedures.

William would also go and sit by the administrator's office and wait for his responses to him during the day, attempting to develop an employee client relationship with upper level management. It is the development of these types of relationships that enhance the quality of life for individuals with disabilities in long-term care facilities; improving quality of care and customer satisfaction.

Effective Management

Basic management skills of problem solving, decision making, planning, delegation, effective communication, meeting -management and self-management are a necessity for any individual in a middle management position in long-term care structure. People management skills are also a required skill set for individuals employed in middle management positions within the long-term care environment. Administrators and Director of Nurses in the nursing home setting encounter many different cultural beliefs, ethnicities, personalities, and communication patterns with both employees and customers in the work environment. Effectively communicating with individuals in long-term care facilities assists with the formulation of purposeful team work, increased staff morale, and decreased employee turnover; resulting in improved quality of services delivered to clients in the nursing homes throughout the nation.

To communicate effectively managers need to express their ideas and thoughts clearly and concisely; encouraging feedback from employees to enhance understanding and retention of messages delivered in the long-term care setting. Effective communication skills also require an ability to manage conflict by exposing problems and collaborating to resolve conflictive dynamics in the work environment; assisting in maintaining equilibrium and stability with employee relations. Healthy communication patterns and positive conflict resolution skills demonstrated by leaders in the work environment sets an example of "acceptable norms" for employee behaviors; middle management leading by setting positive communication examples is a very effective strategy in the long-term care industry when supported by senior level management within nursing home facilities.

All employees in a nursing home environment need to psychologically perceive the unit as a team working towards the same goals for improvement and maintenance of quality of services rendered for an institution to work effectively. Teambuilding requires effective management strategies to psychologically formulate positive and productive teams in the long-term care environment. Some examples for positive psychological team-building include —

- Rewarding Team Successes
- Utilizing Team Meetings
- Rewarding Individual Successes
- Setting Goals of Teamwork
- Building on Individual and Team Self-Esteem
- Formulating & Utilizing Team Newsletters

Teambuilding is an essential component in the long-term care industry. Negative attitudes demonstrated by employees deter an ability to formulate effective teams, positive outcomes for corporations, and sustained quality of care delivered to the elderly in our nation. When negative attitudes are displayed by subordinates in nursing home environments a manager can attempt to change the attitude by example leading; but, unfortunately at times this does not work and termination of relationships is a necessity to accomplish the mission and vision of the specific institution or corporation.

Attempts to reverse developed negative situations in a nursing home through managing difficult employees may require a numerous amount of behavioral strategies utilized by middle management. It is very important to remember not to engage in a battle of the egos with a negative individual; anger feeds anger, and negativity spreads within an institution when ego battlefields develop in the work environment. Difficult employees are generally focused on their own agenda and needs in the employment setting; not team, client, or corporate needs and goals. Explaining the reason base why difficult employees will generate drama in the work environment for their own personal gain.

Middle managers that have effective communication skills possess an ability to be descriptive about behaviors displayed to an employee; defining clear, concise, and objective directions about expectations for improvement within the business environment. Documentation is a very important part of the management process; effective documentation should be thorough, focused on behaviors and quality of work performed; demonstrating objective not subjective observations and evaluations of an employee. Middle managers need to —

- Know what is under their control
- Remember who they are dealing with
- Prepare for the worst
- Not reward inappropriate behavior
- Keep conversations as neutral as possible

The following case demonstrates how assessment and evaluation strategies work in the long-term care industry. Unfortunately, negative incidents do happen from time to time with employees and elaborating on this next case demonstrates how middle management handles negative encounters in the nursing home environment.

A very large facility housing approximately 240 beds had an incident occur with the stealing of narcotics by an employee. The situation transpired as follows:

> A specific LPN worked on a Friday afternoon and counted narcotics with the oncoming shift prior to having the weekend off. When the nurse returned to work on Monday morning, she realized that something was dramatically wrong with the narcotic count. The number of medications (pills) in the cassettes matched the numbers that were written on the narcotic sheets, but they were dramatically off in numbers by comparison to Friday afternoons count. The LPN reported this observation to the Director of Nursing in the facility.

> A nurse manager conversed with the LPN to get an idea of the number of narcotics that were present on Friday versus what was available on Monday morning.

Medication records were reviewed to get an accurate assessment of the number of narcotics administered over the weekend.

Pharmacy was contacted to obtain an accurate number of the narcotics dispensed to the facility for the particular patients in question.

A conclusion was reached that approximately four patients had narcotics missing ranging from 8–20 pills for each patient. At this point the administrator was notified of the narcotics discrepancy within the facility. The administrator of this particular facility instructed a staff member to call in every employee that passed medications over the weekend for an interview and urinalysis test, and notified corporate management of the narcotics discrepancy. Phone calls were made to suspected staff by the Director of Nursing, and every employee complied with the administrators request except one.

One medication aide had suddenly moved and relocated to another state. A conclusion was reached that this particular medication aide had stolen the narcotics, and then shredded the old narcotic sheets after rewriting them to make the number of pills in the cassettes coincide with the numbers documented on the narcotic ledgers. Obviously stated, the medication aide was turned into the state Health and Human Services Department, reports were written and filed with corporate headquarters and required state entities to ensure the medication aide would not practice in any other facility in the state.

Middle management employees in the nursing home structure will implement processes to protect clients from adversities in the long-term care industry, sustaining quality of services delivered through eradication of problematic individuals in the profession.

According to the Management and Business Administration, effective management includes an ability to assess the institutions internal and external structures / dynamics within the work environment. This strategy includes middle managers effectively evaluating —

Strengths	*Weaknesses*
Opportunities	*Threats*

Dynamics surrounding strengths, opportunities, weaknesses and threats assist in establishing goal setting and calculating percentages of success with obtaining specified goals for a nursing home; setting the groundwork for positive outcomes with services rendered. An example of utilizing this strategy in the long-term care industry is as follows —

Strengths:

> *Strong rehabilitation team*
> *Competitive room occupancy cost factor*
> *Positive survey results*
> *Effective networking in medical community*

Weaknesses:

> *Moderate staff turnover*
> *Lack of adequate leadership*
> *Decrease RN employment accessibility*
> *Poor community involvement*
> *Decreased staff morale*

Opportunities:

> *Remodeling or restructuring building*
> *Improving tracking systems*
> *Certification of nurses*
> *Unfulfilled customer needs*
> *New products, systems, technology*

Threats:

> *Shift in Consumer perception of facility &services*
> *Competitive corporations & nursing homes in region*
> *New regulatory guidelines and survey processes*

Various combinations of strategies can be utilized with this process:

- Strength & Opportunity strategies utilize opportunities that maximize the institutions strengths.

- Weakness & Opportunity strategies overcome the institutions weaknesses to pursue current opportunities.

- Strength & Threat strategies identify ways that an institution can utilize its strengths to decrease potential of harm from threats.

- Weakness & Threat strategies set in action mechanisms and dynamics to prevent an institution's weaknesses from making it a target to threats.

Effectively performing these evaluations in the right combination within nursing home institutions will increase the probability
rate for success with services delivered, improving stability of corporations in the long-term care industry.

Management strategies are required with the admission assessment process within long-term care facilities. Client population,
staffing ratios, staff training, and services delivered are all factors to
consider with the potential admission process. A situation encompassing a 35 year old man being assessed while residing on a psychiatric ward for potential admission to a nursing home that was
diagnosed with Korsakoff's syndrome, demonstrates the potential
diversity of nursing home clients within the industry.

Steve's story

Steve was admitted to a psychiatric facility because of inappropriate social behaviors and being a danger to himself due
to his mental decline. Steve's psychological problems were related to thiamine deficiency in the brain resulting from alcohol
consumption, leading to destruction of brain cells and subsequently his diagnosis of Korsakoff's syndrome; which left him
unable to take care of himself without professional healthcare
assistance.

A nurse stated, "It was so sad to watch Steve; his distorted
mannerisms, erratic speech, loss of balance, and inability to
conceptualize his own disturbances."

Steve at the age of 35 had destroyed his health and could no
longer live without healthcare assistance, due to alcoholism.
Steve was not accepted for placement in the nursing home as
he would not have been a good social fit in that specific facility. Steve needed a facility placement that housed some other
young clients to ensure a healthy social environment for him.

Steve is just one example of the diversity of clients assessed for
placement and housed in long-term care facilities. Most individuals
think of long-term care as facilities that only encompass housing for
the elderly, yet there can be a wide range of client ages, diagnosis,
prognosis, stay periods, and treatments. Nursing Homes are not facilities as the psychological perception prevails in society for the el-

derly population to visit prior to death; long-term care facilities are institutions that provide as stated long-term care or in many cases short-term care for all individuals in need of their services within society.

Director Of Nursing

A Director of Nursing position in the long-term care industry can be a rewarding challenge for any nurse that desires to see the quality of services rendered to our elderly be developed, improved, and sustained in nursing home structure. The lead nursing management position requires primary job functions of planning, coordinating and managing patient care services departments including, but not limited to the nursing department to obtain and sustain the highest quality of healthcare for clients within the industry. Responsibilities for a Director of Nurses in the nursing home environment include, but are not limited to —

- Participating in policy and procedure development that support nursing services objectives providing a favorable physical, social and emotional environment for clients.
- Coordinating and presenting continuing education for staff including changes in the Nurse Practice Act.
- Developing programs for recruitment and retention of staff.
- Providing a supervisory leadership role to staff.
- Demonstrating organization and delegation as required.
- Implementing and participating in meetings to address quality of care and quality assurance in the facility, including proactive systems to decrease negative quality of care dynamics.
- Evaluation of acuity levels ensuring staff / patient ratio for the provision of resident care.
- Effectively communicating in verbal and written forms.
- Developing a nursing department budget and utilizing it effectively.
- Coordinating nursing activities with consultants and other department heads.
- Ensuring compliance with federal, state, local standards and regulations by conducting self-surveys and correcting areas of non-compliance.

- Maintaining cohesive public and professional relationships with clients, families, physicians and the community.
- Assuming full responsibility for the operation and management of the facility in the temporary absence of the administrator.

Most corporations will provide training seminars for nurses to prepare an employee for a Director of Nursing position, whether state or corporate presented the classes do provide an individual with tools necessary to be successful in this position within the long-term care industry. Some corporations have nurses in their DNS positions perform a required computerized test to evaluate knowledge base and intelligence status for performing the lead nurse job requirements. This in and of itself is not a bad idea to ensure an individual is intellectually capable of handling a position that requires taking care of human beings within the medical profession and long-term care arena.

Some of the statements made by clients in the long-term care industry are the elements that keep individuals interested in this aspect of the nursing profession and wanting to continue with strategies to improve their quality of life and care levels. Orval's is one of those stories that depicts the clients' sense of humor.

Orval's story

The nurse stated, "It was so cute. I had gone into the shower room to assess and dress the client's foot due to a pressure ulcer development. The shower room floor was still wet and as I was bending down to measure the wound, my shoes and dress were getting wet in the process."

Nurse: *"I don't know Orval, but I think we are going to have a shower together today."*

Orval sat up in his chair, smiled and announced, *"Well! I am 96 years old and I have never showered with a woman before!"*

Everyone in the shower room started laughing, including Orval. It made the patients' day and the staff's; Orval went around in the facility telling other residents about his humor with the nurse in the shower room, including others in the fun. It is this aspect of the elderly client persona that makes any given day special and makes it a joy to care for them in the industry.

Directors of Nursing, if performing their duties effectively, will put in many hours. Department heads whether they are nursing, administration, dietary, etc., need to be out of their offices and on the floor overseeing and evaluating the level of services provided in a facility to ensure a delivery of high level quality care. Sitting behind a desk doing paper work eight or more hours a day does not produce an environment conducive for high level patient care in the healthcare continuum within the medical profession.

The Director of Nursing position can be a very strenuous position in the long-term care arena. A nurse in this position requires the assistance and support of an administrator to accomplish the goal of high client healthcare deliverance and customer perceived satisfaction with healthcare delivery systems. Obtaining any objective in a business setting requires a team of individuals with the same focus, vision and mission; including the medical profession.

The long-term care industry is no different than any other business surrounding this perspective. There is a requirement for customer satisfaction, high level deliverance of services and monetary objectives met to sustain operational standards of a corporation and facilities within the nation. Middle management employee positions are the entities that hold the most responsibility for meeting these objectives in the long-term care industry.

Quality assurance meetings should be held weekly evaluating percentage ratings in a facility concerning pressure ulcers, skin tears, bruises, falls, weight loss, restraints: chemical & physical, fractures, medication errors, infections and psychotropic medications. During these meetings ratios need to be evaluated and proactive interventions formulated and implemented to decrease the ratio numbers with current and future clients. A nursing department being proactive in prevention with deliverance of services rendered will institute a psychology surrounding the development of high level care delivery systems in a facility. Motivating line staff to participate in a proactive preventative intervention psychology will increase the potential of success in nursing home facilities within the long-term care industry. Adjunct services and consultants in-cluding pharmacists, dietitians, occupational therapists, physical therapists, speech pathologists, beauticians, barbers, hospice pro-viders, physicians, and nurse consultants should be included in the goals and focus of a facility's delivery systems to ensure compliance in their services rendered within nursing homes in the nation.

Customer (family or client) complaints are an aspect of the Di-rector of Nursing job requirements that encompass problem solving skills and creative thinking processes to ensure positive relation-ships and customer satisfaction in the long-term care industry. All complaints need to be listened to, taken seriously, and acted on to ensure high level satisfaction with the customer in a nursing home setting. Unmet needs can psychologically trigger increased behav-iors in individuals, generating a cycle of dissatisfaction and contin-ued complaints in a work environment and potentially formulating a negative psychological perception within the industry. The fol-lowing case depicts a new Director of Nursing involved with a situ-ation surrounding customer complaints in a facility due to eradica-tion of side rails in the institution.

In the 1990s, educational processes were initiated about side rail utilization as a restraint, and unsafe practices resulting in 200–300 deaths from side rail utilization in the nation over an approximately 15 year time span. What was psychologically thought to be an in-tervention for safety was proving to be detrimental for the geronto-logical clientele.

The Director of Nursing proceeded with interventions, encom-passing the slow removal of all side rails in the facility where she was practicing nursing, to improve quality of care for the clients.

Some of the customers (family members) did not share her view and felt the DNS was creating an unsafe environment for their loved ones.

In hindsight, the nurse learned that she should have had a family meeting to explain the rationale for side rail removal and provide educational processes to assist individuals to understand the reason base for eradication as a safety intervention within current nursing practice. Family members will not always accept decisions based on a nurses educational levels and knowledge base about geron-tological nursing within the long-term care industry. No citation was issued over the situation, because the nurse was attempting to improve quality of care services delivered in the facility; yet the entire process did create an avenue for educational interventions with clients, family members, staff, and state surveyors to improve quality of care services within a facility.

Assistant Director of Nursing

An Assistant Director of Nursing is utilized in most facilities over 60 beds. This nursing job is an important management po-sition, as the person assists the Director of Nursing Services in managing the licensed and non-licensed employees who provide services and healthcare to clients in a long-term care facility. The Assistant Director of Nursing position reports directly to the DNS, and compliments the Director of Nursing in planning, developing, implementing, and supervising activities in the nursing department including —

Nursing Services Objectives
Policies and Procedures
Disciplinary Action
Hiring and Terminating Staff
Guidelines in accordance with state and federal regulations.

An Assistant Director of Nursing assists with observation and evaluation of care delivery systems through monitoring nursing ac-tivities in a long-term care facility. Dave's case demonstrates how simple gestures performed by an ADNS can change psychological perceptions within the industry.

Dave's story

Dave was a large gentleman diagnosed with cardiac problems, placed in isolation due to airborne MRSA (methicillin resis-tant staphylococcus aureus) and had developed pressure ul-cers from another institution. Dave's son who was a minister flew in from Europe to visit his father, due to the decline in his condition. Family members were a little upset because of their father's condition and potentially rightfully so, but the pressure

ulcer development did not occur in the facility Dave was currently residing in within the industry.

Nurse: "*I knew I had to do something to decrease the complaints com-
ing from Dave's family. I couldn't change Dave's physical condition right
away, if ever, but I could ensure extra provided care was given to Dave
during his stay.*"

Dave's nails were very long, since nail-trimming service was
not provided in his previous living environment. So, the nurse
decided while the son was visiting, she would go into the room
and trim his nails, shave him, and perform oral hygiene, hoping
this would demonstrate to the family that the facility staff did
want to see quality care services delivered to their loved one.
However, Dave would not allow the nurse to trim either fifth
digit nail, and he was adamant about it.

Dave stated: "*I need those nails for picking my nose.*"

As a professional, the nurse simply complied with Dave's wish-
es and did not make an issue of the request, leaving the fifth
digit nail intact on each hand. The son just smiled and shook
his head. But, this simple gesture of demonstrating a desire to
please Dave and his family did change their perception of the
facility.

Unfortunately, Dave did pass a few days later, but his last couple
of days were filled with compassion from his family, not complaints
about care delivery services. For a nurse in a long-term care facility, prioritizing services rendered is a requirement while managing
patient care loads; end-of-life dynamics should encompass tender
loving care in every aspect of services delivered to the client and
family system.

In the absence of the Director of Nursing Services, an Assistant
Director of Nursing Services will assume the duties of the Director within the long-term care environment. Accountabilities for an
ADNS position include assisting with overseeing clinical operations through incorporating the design, implementation and evaluation of nursing systems. An ADNS should provide reports to the
DNS in regards to operations in the nursing department and assist
in conducting staff meetings as needed in the employment arena.
A nurse in this position must possess supervisory skills and medi-

cal knowledge base to ensure clients are free from abuse, mistreatment, and neglect. An Assistant Director of Nursing also performs educational processes as required to maintain nursing staff awareness and compliance with federal and state regulations relative to resident's rights. In general, an Assistant Director of Nursing will perform the duties required in the nursing department to assist the Director of Nursing with incorporation of an effective productive healthcare delivery system.

Continuing education for staff is a required job function in an ADNS or DNS employment job description. In-services should be provided on a monthly basis to ensure state and federal mandated regulations are met in a facility. Creative thinking processes to promote humor with the educational process can be instituted at times to improve learning and retention. Implementing creative strategies to assist staff in the learning curve could be utilized as follows:

> An in-service on customer service encompassed a skit based on client complaints to demonstrate to staff how they were perceived by the client in the nursing home environment. Three staff participated in the skit; two portrayed as nurse aides and one portrayed as a patient. The nurse aides were getting the patient up in the morning to go to breakfast.
>
> One nurse aide stated: "Sue, did you go to that party last night?"
>
> The other nurse aide replied, "Yea! Did you get a look at Scott? Man is he hot!"
>
> The first aide stated: "Yea, I can't believe that Mary girl was all over him."
>
> The nurse aides continued their conversation about the party while assisting the client, never once conversed with the client, put her shirt on backwards, moved her like a sack of potatoes, put her shoes on the wrong feet, and performed no grooming prior to taking her out for breakfast. The skit was hilarious; everyone laughed loudly during the performance

At the termination of the in-service the nurses educated staff that the dynamics were actual situations that transpired in the facility and the perceptions were the perceptions of actual clients housed in the nursing home. Psychologically, the in-service made staff stop and think about what they actually sounded and looked like to a client while caring for them, improving customer service through demonstrated psychological perceptions and utilization of humor within the educational presentations.

Focus

Middle management positions in the long-term care industry are the aspects in the healthcare continuum that implement strategies and systems to sustain quality of services delivered in a nursing home facility. Senior level management will provide some of the tools to utilize for maintenance or improvement of healthcare delivery systems, but the Administrator and Director of Nursing are responsible for ensuring the tools are utilized effectively in the management capacity position through effective communication, teambuilding, supervision of subordinates, assessment skills, implementing systems and psychologically following the mission and vision of the corporate institution.

Responsibilities increase with each career step up in the healthcare arena. Physical tasks may not be as strenuous as a nurse aide position; but the intellectual requirements, time factor, management strategies, prioritizing abilities, and nursing knowledge base needed for a middle management position far exceed any other nurse position in the long-term care arena. Individuals in the healthcare industry and society need to realize that most management healthcare workers do have the client's best interest at heart and work very hard to accomplish goals of high quality care delivery systems in the long-term care industry.

Developing respect for individuals in middle management positions can be a learned process for subordinate employees and customers, and as a society we need to continue to support this industry with the improvement of healthcare systems in nursing homes within the nation.

CHAPTER THREE. GERONTOLOGICAL NURSING

Gerontology is the scientific study of aging and its effects on the human body including biological, psychological, and sociological phenomena that are associated with old age and aging. Gerontological nursing is an evidence-based practice which addresses needs associated with the aging process of human life, including:

Physiological	*Psychosocial*
Developmental	*Economic*
Cultural	*Spiritual Dynamics*

The gerontological nursing practice encompasses a relationship-centered goal philosophy contributing to healthy aging processes for individuals through encouraging developmental well-being in the elderly; assisting clients to adapt to physical and social changes during a life span. The concept of encouraging developmental well-being in the geriatric nursing spectrum assists in and often leads to the interdisciplinary and multi-agency care of our elderly in the nation. Gerontological nursing may be practiced in a variety of settings, but is most likely developed in areas that specialize in the care of elderly clients such as long-term care facilities, assisted living facilities, and sub-acute units within the medical profession.

Assisting in the vision and goals of improving care delivery systems for elderly clients is the Gerontological Nursing Interventions Research Center (GNIRC) which strengthens and expands intervention focused research concerning gerontological nursing and related disciplines through examining and studying the health of elders in a variety of care settings. The GNIRC institute leads research to improve the quality of life for the geriatric population in the United States. Current regions being explored in the revision process surrounding nursing scope of practice standards include:

- Recognition of assumptions with aging as a motivating force in the approach and philosophy of care delivery systems.
- Renewing awareness of the increasing aging population in the nation.
- Identifying barriers caused by stereotypes and myths concerning the aging process.
- The need of a requirement to institute models of care in the geriatric profession.
- Acknowledging diversity of groups and the need for cultural competence within gerontological care.

A new topic of study called ethnogeriatrics addresses cultural competence in the specialty area of gerontology; placing emphasis on the intersect of knowledge from the fields of aging, health, and ethnicity. It is widely accepted that cultural beliefs and practices influence a client's health, behavior, utilization of health care services, client-clinician relationship, and clinician interaction with geriatric clients in the healthcare continuum. The field of ethnogeriatrics will continue to evolve and expand over time with the collection of data and research; assisting in the improvement of care delivery systems for gerontological clients in the nation.

Gerontological Nurses

Nurses that choose the geriatric spectrum for their practice must possess knowledge, skills, and experience surrounding gerontological nursing including a commitment to a vision for improvement and maintenance of quality care delivery systems. Gerontological nurses are healthcare professionals that are responsible for care of geriatric clients across clinical settings and leading inter-professional teams in a holistic person centered approach with delivery of healthcare systems for the geriatric population in the medical community. These nurses work jointly with elderly clients and their families in a client's life span addressing goals in the areas of —

Autonomy

Health

Activities of daily living

Comfort and quality of life during the aging and dying processes

Geriatric nurses assess client health dynamics; develop and implement client care plans; maintain medical records; administer nursing care to ill, injured, convalescent or disabled clients; and may advise on health maintenance and disease prevention or provide case management in the nursing profession. Utilization of the nursing process; an individualized problem solving approach to the nursing care of clients that includes four stages: assessment, planning, implementation, and evaluation is encompassed in gerontological nursing within the medical profession. The nursing process is an essential methodology to identify and measure the outcome of goals implemented with geriatric clients within the healthcare continuum.

Gerontological Nurse, RN, C indicates a specialization in providing nursing care for the geriatric population. A specialized RN, C also entails the responsibility of assisting to improve health and prevent possible consequences of chronic disease, while involving the client and family in educational processes. Certification of nursing practice signifies attainment of a specific criterion involving knowledge, skills, and abilities in a specific specialty field; certified nurse's currently comprise a minority of the professional nurse population. Gerontological certification is valid for three years and requires renewal through a process of met criteria by the nurse within the specialty area of practice in the medical profession.

The American Nurse Credentialing Center (ANCC), a subsidiary of the American Nurses Association (ANA) assists with the achievement of practice excellence through certification of nurses in gerontological nursing. The organization also recognizes healthcare organizations by promoting safe positive work environments through the Magnet Recognition Program and The Pathway to Excellence Program. The ANCC also accredits providers of continuing education programs, provides information and educational services/products to support its care credentialing programs within the nursing profession.

A clinical nurse specialist in gerontology or genomics (study of genes and their function) is defined as a clinical nurse that performs in emerging roles encompassing genetics and its effects on the care of seniors and their families. The field of genomics is advancing the understanding of the aging process and the onset of chronic illnesses within the nation. As this specialty gains more insight about the aging process and gene function concerning diseases; gerontology and geriatric practice theory surrounding the scope of nursing will adapt to their contributions to the medical profession.

The Hartford Institute for Geriatric Nursing was developed in 1996 with funding from the John A. Hartford foundation. It encompasses a mission of improving the quality of care for the elderly within the nation through demonstrated gerontological competence with nurses in the medical profession. Geriatric nursing is a major structure surrounding the New York University College of Nursing program, and the Hartford Institute is a key element for structuring the philosophies and educational resources for this nursing program. The college offers Masters and Post-Masters programs for nurses interested in Geriatric Nurse Practitioners (GNP) careers within the nursing profession. Several programs and projects have been initiated by the Hartford Institute including —

- Geriatric competence of specialty nurses: REASN – Resourcefully Enhancing Aging in Specialty Nursing.
- NICHE – Nurses Improving Care Health Systems for Elders.
- Hartford Institute partnership with the American Association of Colleges of Nursing.
- Coalition of geriatric nursing organizations.
- Consortium of New York Geriatric Education Center.
- Culture change: nursing homes as clinical training sites.
- Preparing nurse faculty to supervise student rotations in care of older adults.
- Geriatric nursing competency in home care.

- The Geriatric Interdisciplinary Team training project.
- Geriatric nursing summer scholars and fellows program.
- Developmental research on elder mistreatment.
- Training of advanced practice nurses in geriatrics.
- Enhancing nurse competence in care for older adults.

Sam's case demonstrates the essential requirement for understanding and educational knowledge base concerning behaviors and psychology surrounding the geriatric population.

Sam's story

Sam had resided in the same nursing home for several years and had demonstrated no psychological dysfunction during the previous years.

Sam was sitting on the side of his bed, watching television, when the geriatric nurse entered Sam's room.

The geriatric nurse removed Sam's shoe and sock, and began to assess Sam's wound after removal of the dressing.

Looking up after the dressing removal to converse with Sam the nurse noticed Sam was placing his penis in a glass of milk, coaxing his penis to drink.

Sam had developed a disease process that interfered with his body chemistry, resulting in Sam acquiring a psychology of viewing his penis as a baby. On the following day, Sam was sitting in the dining room attempting to feed his penis a sandwich. Blood chemistries drawn revealed the discrepancy generating psychological difficulties for the client; when chemistry levels were returned to normal, Sam's distorted psychology was re-balanced, and Sam returned to his normal routine of functions within the nursing home environment.

This particular situation demonstrates the nurse requirement of knowledge base that chemistry alterations concerning gerontological clients can manifest psychological symptomology.

The following diagram demonstrates the chain of command in the long-term care nursing department.

CHAIN OF COMMAND

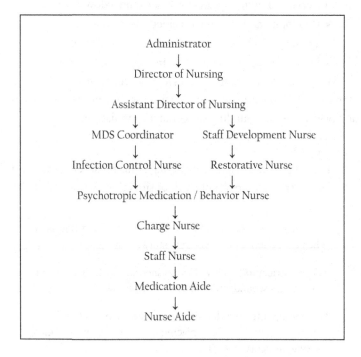

Registered Nurses

A registered nurse is an individual that is educated in the scientific basis of nursing, and meets certain prescribed standards of knowledge base and clinical competence within the medical profession. Registered nurses are healthcare professionals responsible for implementing the practice of nursing through utilization of the nursing process in conjunction with other healthcare professionals. The healthcare profession requires registered nurses to be client advocates through instilling nursing processes of assessment, planning, implementation, and evaluating nursing care of the ill and injured within the healthcare continuum. Registered nurses regardless of their nursing specialty or work setting: treat patients, educate patients, educate the public about various medical conditions, and provide advice / emotional support to patients' and family members within their specific region of practice.

Registered nurses are the largest group of healthcare workers; comprising approximately 2.5 million active employees in the workforce. An educational degree is an essential job requirement for a registered nurse and may be any of the following: Bachelor of Science in Nursing (BSN), Associate Degree in Nursing (ADN), or a diploma degree obtained from an accredited school of nursing. Successful completion of the NCLEX-RN examination is mandated prior to active practice in any field of nursing. Advanced practice nurses that require a master's degree include —

Clinical Nurse Specialists	*Nurse Anesthetists*
Nurse Midwives	*Nurse Practitioners*

Bachelor of Science degrees in nursing programs are offered by colleges or universities and require four years for completion of a nursing program. Associate Degree in nursing programs are offered by community or junior colleges and require two to three years of educational processes to graduate and be eligible for NCLEX testing. Diploma programs are offered in hospitals and consist of a three year study curriculum. Accelerated master degree programs typically take three to four years to complete and nurses with a Bachelor's Degree may enter these programs within the nation.

Scope of practice is determined by each state's Nurse Practice Act. A registered nurses scope of practice can be very broad and differentiate from state to state, and institution to institution. Nurse Practice Acts will —

Outline legal practice for a registered nurse

Direct nurses on tasks performed or not performed with a specific practice

All registered nurses should be caring, sympathetic, responsible, and detail oriented within their specific practice in the medical profession. Registered nurses must possess emotional stability, eliciting an ability to cope with the demands and stresses of the profession; such as human suffering and emergencies. Intellect of a registered nurse determines their ability to correctly assess patient's conditions and establish the requirement for additional medical consultation in the nursing profession.

All long-term care facilities are required by regulatory guidelines to provide licensed nursing services twenty-four hours per day seven days per week. Registered nurses are mandated by federal regulations to be in skilled nursing home facilities at least eight consecutive hours per day seven days per week. One registered nurse needs to be designated as a Director of Nursing in the nursing home structure on a fulltime basis to conform to federally mandated regulations governing long-term care facilities within the nation.

Licensed Practical Nurses

Nurses in LPN positions within the medical profession are individuals that have completed a practical nursing program and are licensed by a state to provide routine patient care under the direction of a registered nurse or a physician. Licensed Practical Nurses (LPN'S) have the technical knowledge base to perform routine nursing duties, manage clerical duties and maintain records in the nursing profession. A main responsibility of the LPN job is to accept and implement orders from qualified professionals on a team that are authorized to independently diagnosis and treat patients. Licensed Practical nurses are the healthcare providers that deliver direct basic patient care to clients in the medical profession. Successful completion of the NCLEX-LPN is a necessity prior to active nursing practice in any venue within the medical profession. Some states will refer to these nurses as Licensed Vocational Nurses in the healthcare continuum.

Educational requirements for an LPN consist of a one year program offered at community colleges, technical and vocational schools, and some hospitals in the nation. Admission into an LPN program usually requires a high school degree, passing an aptitude test, and a physical examination prior to acceptance into any program in the United States.

Scope of practice for an LPN is more restrictive than that for an RN; licensed practical nurses are required to work under the direction and supervision of a —

Physician	*Dentist*
Psychologist	*Optometrist*
Nurse Practitioner	*Podiatrist*
Homeopath	*Registered Nurse*

The LPN's scope of practice will vary from state to state, institution to institution, and also varies based on the specific training of the individual nurse within the medical profession. Common tasks that could be performed by an LPN include —

> *Collecting data on patients status*
> *Reporting data*
> *Assist with nursing plan of care and diagnosis*
> *Assist in the implementation of the plan of care*

The LPN must possess innovative mental processes assisting in the capacity to develop strategic interventions while dealing with and handling some geriatric clients in the nursing home environment. Michael's scenario depicts this strategy.

Michael's story

Michael was diagnosed with mixed dementia which generated some difficulties in performing basic hygiene requirements, such as bathing. Michael had refused a bath for approximately two weeks and staff needed to be innovative in their thinking processes to get the task accomplished within the facility. One LPN addressed the dynamic as follows —

Nurse: "Michael, we have a new shower massage. I was wondering if you would like to be the first to try it out?"

Michael: "I don't know."

Nurse: "It will relax your muscles."

Michael: "Will it help my back?"

Nurse: "Yes, it very well could help with your back discomfort."

Michael complied with the nurse's request and tried the shower massage, and his lack of hygiene practices were addressed through innovative thinking on the part of his nurses.

LPNs with demonstrated higher intellectual levels may advance their skill set in the medical profession. An LPN-C is an LPN that is specifically trained in intravenous therapy; possessing basic skill proficiency and knowledge to perform the function competently and safely. LPN'S in general may observe and monitor IV fluid administration, calculate and maintain flow rates of infusions, discontinue IV infusions, and report/document observation and procedures concerning IV therapy. LPN-Cs under the direct supervision and direction of a registered nurse, physician or dentist may —

- Perform venipuncture to initiate the administration of IV fluid via peripheral veins.
- Change or add parental solutions to existing IV lines.
- Change IV tubing and dressings.
- Add to existing IV lines premixed medications.
- Maintain the patency of heparin locks.

Charge Nurses

Charge nurses are individuals in the long-term care setting that are responsible for independent supervision surrounding delivery of care standards to a group of residents in a nursing unit. These nurses will render professional nursing services in support of medical care and the interdisciplinary team, surrounding the scope of procedures and policies in a particular institution. Duties of a charge nurse can include, but are not limited to:

Assessing resident needs.
Developing individual care plans.
Administering nursing care.
Evaluating nursing care.
Supervising certified nursing assistants, medication aides, LPNs and RNs.
Transcribing and carrying out physician orders as appropriate.
Administering and documenting medications as ordered.
Assisting physicians as necessary.
Recording and reporting appropriate conditions and reactions of patients.

Charge nurses must possess clinical experience, education, and skills specifically to their region of practice. A charge nurse in the long-term care industry is generally a registered nurse. Gerontological charge nurses are required to possess knowledge base of state / federal rules and regulations governing long-term care facilities. Continuing education is a renewal license requirement in the areas of clinical subject, management, personal growth and development within the healthcare continuum. Gerontological charge nurses must demonstrate knowledge of the aging process, possess the ability to assess the client's age specific needs, and provide care as directed by the policies and procedures of a specific facility or organization. An ability to prioritize appropriately and make sound nursing judgments is a necessity for a charge nurse position in the long-term care industry. Secondary functions and skills that may be required for a charge nurse include—

Implementing rehabilitative nursing techniques.
Participating in unit in-service programs.
Maintaining a safe and comfortable working environment.
Basic computer knowledge and ability.
Demonstrating a working knowledge base of infection control practices and principles.

Staff Nurses

Staff nurses provide direct nursing care to clients and assist in the supervision of certified nursing assistants. Staff nurses must also maintain a basic knowledge of state and federal regulations governing long-term care facilities to ensure appropriate healthcare services delivered to clients in the nursing home setting. Essential staff nurse duties may include —

Charting and Documentation Medication Administration
Nursing Care Functions Treatment Administration
Safety and Sanitation Duties
Infection Control Practices
Care Plan Formulation and Implementation(providing assistance)

A nurse in a staff position within the long-term care industry can be an LPN or an RN. Staff nurses are required to maintain adequate physical and sensory requirements in order to be able to perform appropriately in a nursing home setting. Nurses in a staff nurse position must be able to physically move intermittently throughout the day, demonstrate an ability to cope with mental and emotional stress, possess adequate vision and hearing, and must be in generally good health. Front line nurses are required to demonstrate an ability to function independently; possess flexibility; display personal integrity; and work effectively with residents, personnel, and support agencies in the healthcare continuum. A staff nurse is required to relate to and work with the ill, disabled, elderly, emotionally upset, and at times hostile people in the work environment.

Nurses in all spectrums of the profession have stories about procedure performance in the healthcare setting. The following case depicts the multi-requirement of responsibility for a staff nurse. At times employee healthcare dynamics evolve in the work environment as demonstrated in the following situation.

> While changing a dressing, due to the location of the wound the nurse needed an assistant to hold the client's limb during the treatment process. A very brave nursing assistant offered her expertise for the procedure, not knowing that wounds with developed gangrene will generate a very distinctive horrendous odor.

> The nursing assistant made it through the dressing removal and said, "I have to leave." As the assistant was walking out of the room, the nurse heard a thud.

> Putting the limb down and walking into the hallway the staff nurse discovered the nursing assistant passed out on the floor.

> The nursing assistant was revived and the patient wound was treated, but the incident gave staff something to talk about for the remainder of the night. Sometimes employee healthcare dynamics can require staff nurse assessment, treatment, skills, and knowledge base within the long-term care environment.

Ancillary Nurse Positions

There are many ancillary nurse positions within the long-term care industry that assist with quality assurance strategies in the nursing field specialty. Some of these positions are —

Infection Control Nurse	*Staff Development Nurse*
Restorative Coordinator Nurse	*Skin / Wound Nurse*
MDS (Minimum Data Set) Coordinator	
Psychotropic Medication / Behavior Coordinator	

Ancillary nurse positions should be provided within facilities that house sixty certified beds or more to insure quality services delivered to clients within the facilities.

Infection Control Nurse

Infection control nurses are the individuals responsible for planning, developing, directing, implementing and evaluating infection control and prevention programs within a healthcare setting. This particular nurse supervises infection control services and practices for patients, visitors and staff within a facility. There are many duties and responsibilities within an infection control position that include, but are not limited to —

- Collecting data on infections (labs, cultures, nosocomial.)
- Maintaining documentation of each infection process.
- Conducting rounds to monitor infection control practices.
- Investigating incidents of infection.
- Reporting infection control data to the quality assurance team.
- Implementing strategies to decrease the spread of infection.
- Ensuring availability of needed supplies.
- Preparing and monitoring monthly infection control data.
- Analyzing infection control data monthly and yearly.
- Providing educational meetings and in-services to increase compliance with infection control practices.

In-services on infection control can elicit some interesting responses in nursing home facilities as displayed in the following situation.

> Two infection control nurses provided an in-service and decided for fun that they would dress up as infectious bugs (bacteria and virus bugs) to add some humor into the educational process, hopefully improving learning and retention of the topic.

> The nurses providing the in-service were laughing hard giving the presentation, because no one found humor in the joke; it made the educational process ineffective with the audience.

The fact that line staff did not perceive any humor with the bug deliverance did add a lot of humor in the psychological perceptions of senior level management staff, so some individuals did benefit from the scenario, just not the intended audience. Again, the utilization of humor in the long-term care industry can be beneficial if utilized appropriately to improve quality of care delivery services for the gerontological client in the nursing home environment.

MDS Coordinator

The MDS (minimum data set) coordinator position is a Registered nurse job that encompasses completing the MDS form, accurately assessing patients for documentation purposes, completing patient tracking forms, formulating and updating patient care plans, submitting MDS and tracking forms to the state, assessing and formulating care assessment protocols, and participating in care plan meetings within the long-term care structure. An MDS Coordinator nurse ensures compliance, accuracy, and reliability of the clients chart regarding specific records and processes developed off of the MDS form within the long-term care industry.

The MDS form is an assessment tool utilized in the nursing home setting that evaluates and determines treatment, medical care, restorative care, therapy services, activities of daily living, and patient care levels for clients that reside in long-term care facilities. Sections in this form include —

Activities of Daily Living Assistance	*Balance / Gait*
Assistive Devices	*Therapies*
Range of Motion	*Fall History*
Physical Exams	*Physician Orders*
Restorative Nursing Programs	*Medications*
Treatments & Procedures	*Continence*
Disease Diagnosis	*Cognitive Patterns*
Vision Patterns	*Activity Patterns*
Mood and Behavior	*Skin Condition*
Psychosocial Well-Being	*Dental Status*
Oral / Nutritional Status	

The MDS form is submitted to the state and federal government entities for purposes of Medicare and Medicaid reimbursement, surveyor's utilization of data with facility annual survey processes, calculation of quality of care indicators in a specific facility, and to provide information to insurance companies covering clients in nursing homes. An MDS Coordinator must be an individual that is detail oriented, methodical and maintains data and documents with utmost accuracy.

Restorative Nurse

A Restorative Care Coordinator nurse position manages the Re-storative Therapy Department and Resident Safety Program in accordance with state/federal regulatory guidelines in a nursing home setting. This nursing position encompasses duties in the following areas —

- Planning, developing, coordinating, implementing and evaluating restorative services for residents.
- Maintaining complete and accurate records of all assessments and services provided.
- Weekly documentation
- Medicare Part B documentation
- Monthly documentation
- Educating and training facility staff as required in restorative therapy and deliverance.
- Effectively working with the therapy department to ensure appropriate transitional services provided to clients.
- Participating in the RAI (resident assessment instrument) process, effectively communicating with the MDS Coordinator and therapy services department.
- Planning, developing, coordinating, implementing, and evaluating the resident safety programs-initiates proactive interventions for fall prevention and restraint reduction.
- Attending Medicare and Quality Assurance meetings to report on services rendered, patient compliance and improvement, and statistical data obtained with analyzing processes.

Staff Development Nurse

Nurse Staff Development Coordinator positions in the long-term care industry include duties of scheduling staffing hours, providing educational processes within a facility such as monthly in-services, orientation processes of newly hired employees, and may include quality assurance and some infection control functions. A

Staff Development Coordinator nurse should participate in systems addressing staff morale and improving interdepartmental relations within nursing home structure.

Skin / Wound Nurse

A Skin / Wound Care Nurse is responsible for developing a skin care program that includes assessing skin condition and skin alterations concerning clients in nursing home settings. Physicians, charge nurses and the Director of Nursing are to be notified by the wound nurse of any identified skin discrepancies in long-term care facilities. Additional duties for a wound nurse in nursing home structure are: developing plans of care for at risk and wound care clients, obtaining and implementing orders and treatments for wounds, insuring proactive preventative interventions are in place and functioning appropriately, and evaluating the progress of healing wounds within a nursing home facility. The skin nurse should implement a program that maintains every resident being assessed from head to toe on admission and weekly for any skin alterations to insure prompt and proper treatment for any developed pressure ulcers. Client skin assessments should include:

- Obtaining baseline and weekly measurements of all wounds. (pressure ulcers, incision lines, bruises, lacerations etc...)
- Documenting weekly progress of healing with current treatment modalities.
- Assessing all clients with Stage II to IV pressure ulcers 2x weekly.

Skin Care Programs must contain elements that provide staff development, interdisciplinary collaborations with plans of care, utilization of the nursing process, and educational interventions as required by federal regulations to sustain understanding and compliance with initiatives for skin care programs within a nursing home setting. All services rendered in a skin care program must be in accordance with state and federal regulatory guidelines within the long-term care industry.

Pressure ulcer development can occur in the residential home setting, nursing home environments, assisted living facilities, hospitals or Neurogeriatric units within the nation. Nutritional and physical statuses of clients are contributing factors to the development of pressure ulcers and not all pressure ulcers are avoidable with geriatric clients, sometimes pressure ulcers are unavoidable, due to the client's medical condition and /or nutritional status within the nursing home environment. Elizabeth's case depicts this situation.

Elizabeth's story

Elizabeth had lived in her home for as long as possible — her physical and nutritional decline led her to the healthcare admission process.

Elizabeth's pressure ulcer initiated on her coccyx and was approximately 1cm x 1cm when it was first discovered. By the time Elizabeth was admitted to the nursing home facility, due to nutritional decline her pressure ulcer had extended over her lower back, down to mid-buttocks and across the entire width of her body.

Elizabeth was placed on a specialty mattress with pressured air over four inches thick, had dressing changes performed three times per day, and was placed on a bed rest status to decrease pressure to the wound. A feeding tube was placed prior to nursing home admission to address the nutritional decline status.

It took a year and a half to heal the wound for a surgical closure procedure. Elizabeth was allowed up and out of bed for meals at this point to assist with gastrostomy tube removal.

Psychotropic / Behavior Nurse

Psychotropic Medication / Behavior Nurse Coordinators are the nurses that monitor anti-psychotic, anti-anxiety, and antidepressant medications, while assessing psychiatric patient's behaviors within long-term care facilities to maintain compliance with regulatory guidelines. Nursing homes are federally regulated and mandated to be free of unnecessary physical and chemical restraints within the long-term care environment. A substantiating appropriate diagnosis must be obtained with each antipsychotic medication ordered and the client chart documentation must substantiate that diagnosis. There are only eleven diagnoses that warrant antipsychotic medication utilization within nursing home environments.

Gradual titration (decrease) of all psychotropic medications is recommended unless clinically contraindicated; titrations do not need to be attempted if psychotic features are stabilized with no significant side effects noted from medication utilization with psychiatric clients in nursing homes. Behavior modification programs and daily behavior tracking systems are developed, evaluated, implemented, and monitored by these nurses in accordance with state and federal regulatory guidelines in the nursing home setting. DRR (Drug Regimen Reviews) are conducted by the program nurse, consulting pharmacist, and attending physician on a regular basis to ensure compliance with all psychotropic medications ordered in a long-term care facility. Anti-anxiety and anti-psychotic PRN (as needed) medications also are in the category of required federally mandated evaluation and the psychiatric / behavior nurse should monitor utilization and compliance with titration (decrease) of these medications within a nursing home facility.

The psychiatric nurse performs her duties in collaboration with pharmacists, psychiatrists, and physicians to ensure all psychotropic medications and psychiatric client behavior modification programs are documented and utilized as regulated by The Centers for Medicare and Medicaid Services within the nation. Some states have closed all of the Neurogeriatric units in their region. In these cases, clients diagnosed with psychiatric conditions are placed in long-term care facilities. The following case about a client diagnosed with schizophrenia demonstrates that even a client that is usually lost in delusions and hallucinations can find a moment of clarity to realize that their perceptions are different from others'.

Pat's story

A nurse was conversing with Pat about her displayed behaviors: she appeared more anxious and upset than usual for people in the nursing home environment.

During the conversation Pat stated, "My brain does not work like other people's brains work."

The moment of clarity was brief, and then Pat was lost in another delusion, yet it did demonstrate to the nurse that even individuals with a severe mental illness could be psychologically in reality for brief periods of time. This aspect of gerontological nursing does pose some challenges when managing client care loads and placement standards, but it brings some intellectual challenges that would not be possible without psychiatric diagnosed clients in the nursing home setting within the long-term care profession.

Focus

Gerontological nursing encompasses a varied spectrum of practices within the health care continuum and focuses on the improvement of quality of care for the aging individual in the long-term care industry. Registered nurses and licensed practical nurses that choose this career path usually do so to generate some type of change in the services delivered to the elderly within our nation. Assisting clients through the aging process, and the death and dying process can be a rewarding challenge for healthcare professionals in the medical field.

The variety of diagnosis, medical circumstances, age factors, management strategies, family involvement, and state / federal regulatory changes make this spectrum of the nursing profession an intellectually satisfying challenge for many nurses in the medical profession. As specific regions of research and study surrounding ethnogeriatrics, genomics, and the Gerontological Nursing Interventions Research Center continue to evolve, reveal and release educational information encompassing the aging and dying processes within the lifespan. Gerontonlogical nurses will implement new strategies and interventions into their nursing practice, improving quality of care delivery systems and services for the gerontological population within society and nursing home structure in the long-term care industry.

CHAPTER FOUR. DIRECT CARE PROVIDERS

Certified nursing assistants (CNA'S) are employees in the medical profession that spend the most time with clients, providing basic activity of daily living requirements in healthcare based environments. It is estimated that 70-90% of the direct care services provided to patients is by the nursing assistant within long-term care facilities. Individuals employed in a gerontological CNA position must possess personality traits and psychological processes of compassion, flexibility, respectfulness, integrity, reliability, and a desire to assist the elderly. A nursing assistant position is an entry level role in the health care industry. Several other names are utilized for this position, included but not limited to —

Home Health Aide	*Nursing Assistant*
Patient Care Technician	*Direct Care Provider*

The majority of nursing assistants do possess a desire to learn and please clients under their care. Unfortunately, it is the few individuals that have made headlines in the media that formulate perceptions in society about nursing assistants in long-term care facilities. The reality of the situation is that most direct care providers are kind human beings that enjoy assisting and caring for patients within the health care continuum in the medical profession.

There are many employment opportunities for a certified nursing assistant in areas such as —

Hospitals	*Hospice*
Long-term Care Facilities	*Assisted Living Facilities*
Rehabilitative Institutions	*Intermediate Care Facilities*
Home Health Agencies	*Psychiatric Institutions*
Adult Day Care	

In the CNA position, there is a wide range of specialties for an individual to choose from for employment purposes. The diverse specialty aspect of the direct care giver position offers a wide range of capacities and availabilities to draw individuals into a professional medical career. It is not unusual for individuals to initiate their careers at a CNA entry level position and work their way up the ladder to registered nurses or advance practice nurses within the healthcare continuum.

History of Certified Nursing Assistants

The Volunteer Nurses' Aide Service was the first program developed for nurse aide employment during World War I to assist professional nurses with the impact of casualties, due to the increased need for patient assistance surrounding basic care requirements. Individuals received training from nurses and then were allowed to perform skills that were more tedious and daily required duties of nurses, assisting in rendering adequate healthcare services to the injured and convalescent in hospital settings.

The Ombudsman Reconciliation Act (OBRA) was passed by congress in 1987, due to quality of care and safety concerns in nursing homes within the nation. All Medicare and Medicaid certified nursing home facilities are required to be staffed by well trained personnel under OBRA laws. OBRA regulations, thus initiated the first state certified nursing assistant classes to be formulated in the United States.

In the 1980's, staff performance levels in nursing homes increased with the training of nursing assistants performed by either registered nurses or licensed practical nurses in a formal classroom setting, including theoretical and practical clinical competency testing. There are basic skills that a nursing assistant must be able to perform in any institution within the medical field and OBRA laws govern CNA programs to ensure these basic requirements are met and sustained in the nation. All CNA educational programs are required to be surveyed through the Health and Human Services state survey processes every two years to maintain compliance with regulatory guidelines surrounding nursing assistant training in the medical profession.

Certified Nursing Assistant: Education & Training

A direct care provider has to be at least sixteen years of age and possess the ability to read, write and understand the English language. State certified training programs are offered in long-term care facilities, junior colleges, technical colleges, and Red Cross organizations within the nation. There is a variance on the time factor involved with each specific nursing assistant training program ranging from 76 hours to 120 hours. Completion of a nursing assistant program can take from two to twelve weeks to obtain finalization of training for an individual, depending on each state's regulatory guidelines.

Evaluations by nurses will consist of both written and skill set testing to ensure competency of nursing assistants within the medical profession. A registered nurse must oversee the CNA program and perform the state skill testing portion of the student curriculum. Each program must contain at least sixteen hours of clinical training and one hour of abuse/neglect education for the nursing assistant trainee to meet federal regulatory guidelines in the nation.

After successful completion of a nursing assistant program the student receives a certificate and is eligible to test for certification through a monitored state testing program. Health and Human Services state testing is performed by a registered nurse and consists of a written exam of fifty questions or more, and a skill set testing packet of at least six random skills that must be performed by the student. After successful completion of state testing a certified nursing assistant is then placed on the state registry in the state of employment.

The purpose of a nurse aide registry is to maintain a database of individuals who meet federal requirements to provide care giving to patients in institutions within the medical field. A registry is also a tool utilized in the healthcare field to check certification status of individuals; and findings of abuse, neglect or misappropriation of property, which is a federal mandated requirement prior to employing any individual in the healthcare profession. For each certified nursing assistant the registry contains —

> *Basic identifying information*
> *Care giver work history*
> *Eligibility status for working in the medical field*
> *Findings of abuse, neglect, or misappropriation of property*

The following incident does depict the fact that some nurse aides try very hard to perform a good job taking an opportunity to go the extra mile, yet it does not always transpire as a CNA would hope. A particularly ambitious nursing assistant decided after she had all of her patients in bed for the night that she would mop all the floors in the patient rooms and hallway on her unit.

> The nurse aide filled her bucket with warm water and added the cleanser under the counter in the hopper room — mopped all the floors — gave her report — and went home for the night.

> When she returned to work the next day, housekeeping asked to speak with the nurse aide. The cleanser she had chosen had stripped all the wax off of the floors in the patient rooms and hallway.

Housekeeping was curious to know how it had happened. The chemical used by the certified nursing assistant was not labeled and was incorrectly assumed to be a floor disinfectant. Some staff found humor in the incident and in the nurse aide's ambition, but not the housekeeping department in this particular nursing home.

Since the 1980s, all chemicals are required to be identified properly with labels, and logged on the MSDS (material safety data sheets) through OSHA (Occupational Safety Health Administration) regulatory guidelines in nursing home structure.

Certified Nursing Assistant Duties

A certified nursing assistant position requires the individual to work under direct supervision of a registered nurse or licensed practical nurse in the medical field. Duties range from state to state, institution to institution, and specific training of the direct care provider. Some of the skill sets required are listed below, but may change depending on the type of institution the CNA is employed in and specific training of the CNA —

Dental Hygiene	*Nail Care*
Basic Personal Hygiene	*Bathing and Dressing*
Toileting	*Food Consumption*
Catheter Care	*Vital Signs*
Repositioning	*Transferring*
Answering Call Lights	*Documentation*
Post Mortem Care	*Effective Communication*
Recreational Activities	*Restorative Nursing*
Ambulation	*Reporting*

A position as a certified nursing assistant should not be taken lightly; it is a very important role in the medical field. Nursing assistants are vital to the safety, care, and well-being of clients in any setting within the healthcare continuum. Efficiency of basic care services is sustained with well trained and responsible direct care providers in any institution.

Certified nursing assistants often develop personal connections with their clients, due to the amount of time that they spend caring for individuals in long-term care facilities. It is this aspect of the job that naturally evolves over time that keeps so many direct care providers dedicated to their clients and the institutions that employ them in the nation. An example of CNA dedication to their job and the clients under their care is exemplified in the following case.

> LPN John approached the Director of Nursing in the hallway and stated, "Joan does not feel well. I have tried to get her to go home, but she will not leave her patients."

The Director of Nursing instructed John to bring Joan to her office. After seeing Joan the nurse realized that the CNA was in serious trouble. Joan was holding her chest and complaining of palpitations. Joan relayed to the nurse that she had received triple bypass surgery in the past.

The nurse took Joan's pulse and blood pressure. BP was 210/140. Pulse was 120. They phoned 911 immediately and Joan was taken to the emergency room at the local hospital, admitted to the intensive care unit and placed on a nitroglycerine drip.

> The CNA was more concerned about who would take care of her patients versus her own health, demonstrating the level of dedication some CNAs have concerning their jobs and care of their clients in the long term care industry.

Medication Aide Training

A certified medication aide is a certified nursing assistant who has successfully completed a training program approved by their specific state of employment for medication administration by demonstrating passing scores on written and clinical examinations, and who has obtained certification as a medication aide provided by the state of practice through demonstrated competency on a written examination. Medication Aide classes are offered in technical colleges, vocational colleges, junior colleges, long-term care facilities, and assisted living facilities. There is a variance on the hours involved with a medication aide training class ranging from 48-100 depending on each states regulatory guidelines. To enroll in a medication aide training class an individual must be at least 18 years of age and possess certification as a nursing assistant. Potential students must also be of good moral standing and have no criminal history. A medication aide training program will contain primary educational processes including—

> Basic medication administration, storage, and handling competencies evaluations

> Basic medication procedures

> Supporting medication procedures

> Drug education

Human body system education

> *Musculoskeletal*
> *Urinary*
> *Endocrine*
> *Reproductive*
> *Circulatory*
> *Nervous*
> *Respiratory*
> *Eyes and Ears*
> *Integumentary*

Once medication aide training is complete with passing scores demonstrated, graduates are required to obtain certification through the National Council of State Board of Nursing. Certification testing must be completed within three months of completing a state approved medication aide class. A certified medication aide is required to have ten units of continuing education and recertify every two years to maintain active status through the medication aide registry. A medication aide registry is similar to the certified nursing assistant registry and is utilized for similar purposes within the healthcare profession.

Medication Aide Scope of Practice

Under the supervision of a charge nurse; certified medication aides administer oral, inhalation and topical medications to clients as prescribed by a physician. A medication aide in the long-term care industry is also responsible for —

> *Observing for adverse medication reactions*
> *Reporting any adverse signs or symptoms to the charge nurse*
> *Observing for the effectiveness of medications*
> *Appropriately documenting medication administration times*

All skills performed by a medication aide in the nursing home environment needs to be in accordance with state and federal regulations, current standards of nursing practice, and the policies and procedures of each specific institution. The Medication Aide Act instituted in 1998, legally defines the scope of practice for individuals employed in healthcare that administer medications to patients. The Medication Aide Act states, "The Legislature finds that the administration of medications by persons other than oneself or one's caretaker should be a regulated act and there is a need to define a system to safely assist individuals to take medications who do not have the ability to take medications independently." The purpose of the Act is to ensure health, safety, and welfare of patients by providing for the accurate, efficient, and safe utilization of medication aides to assist in the administration of medications within the healthcare industry.

The routes a medication aide is allowed to administer medications include —

- Oral
- Inhalation
- Topical Instillation (eyes, ears, nose)

There are minimum standards for competence set forth by the Medication Aide Act that include maintaining confidentiality, complying with a patient's right to refuse medications, sustaining hygiene, maintaining current infection control standards, documenting accurately/completely and providing medications according to the five rights. The five rights are —

- The Right Drug
- The Right Time
- The Right Patient
- The Right Dose
- The Right Route

According to the Act, a medication aide must also possess an ability to understand and follow instructions, practice safety in administration of medication procedures, comply with limitations and conditions of their practice, and have knowledge of abuse and neglect reporting requirements within the healthcare profession. A medication aide may also be responsible for additional duties in the long-term care industry that include —

- Proper storage of medications
- Monitoring medications for accountability
- Inspecting and cleaning equipment
- Obtaining accurate vital signs

Focus

Direct care providers are a very integral part of the medical profession. Nurse aides are the team players that spend the majority of time with patients in the long-term care setting and play an important role encompassing the psychosocial and emotional well-being of patients they care for in the industry. Nursing assistant jobs are not to be taken lightly, but viewed as a very serious and important aspect role in quality of care concerning clients in any setting direct care providers are utilized in the medical profession.

Whether it is a certified nurse aide, a medication aide, or both assisting you or your loved one in the long-term care arena try to be appreciative of the effort and cares provided. These individuals do have very demanding jobs that require organizational skills and a lot of patience to meet every client's needs on a daily basis. The truth is that the majority of direct care providers work very hard every day they are employed in their positions in the medical field. Love, kindness, and respect demonstrated by all individuals in healthcare environments while caring for the elderly in our nation will go a long ways to improve the quality of life for residents within the gerontological profession in the nation.

CHAPTER FIVE. PHYSICIAN ROLE

Physicians are an essential component part of the long-term care industry. Clinicians providing services in nursing homes must maintain expertise and knowledge base surrounding —

Acute Medical Care	*Chronic Medical Care*
Infection Control	*Patient Safety*
Abuse Prohibition State	*Regulatory Guidelines*
Federal Regulatory Guidelines	*Medications*
Diagnostic Testing	*Disease Processes Diagnosis*
Disease Processes Treatment	*Professional Standards*
Ethics	*Admission Practices*
Discharge Practices	*Education*
Rehabilitation	
Psychosocial Needs of Patients	

Physicians that demonstrate these standards and knowledge base contribute to the maintenance and improvement of quality of care with clients in nursing home settings within the nation.

With the aging population, a multidisciplinary requirement concerning medical care of clients encompassing a demonstrated expertise of geriatrics, continues the evolvement surrounding quality of care practices with this population within the nation. Physicians, physician assistants, nurse practitioners, and all clinicians in the medical profession need to possess an adequate knowledge base about gerontology, death and dying processes, and general nursing home practices to assist in the process of providing acceptable care levels to the elderly within the United States. In this chapter, we will examine the primary care providers and medical directors' roles in the long term care industry, hopefully expanding the educational knowledge base within society about these roles in the evolving field of gerontology.

Elderly clients in the long term care industry do respect their physicians. New physicians tend to put forth a little more effort in their care delivery services with gerontological clients in nursing home environments. It is interesting to observe new physicians evolve in their careers; building up their client base and developing their reputations within the social and medical community. New physicians generally want to please their patients and gerontological clients do need extra attention at times in the nursing home setting. A new primary care provider usually will assist in meeting some of the geriatric population's psychosocial requirements within the long-term care facilities in the nation.

Medical Directors

Medical Directors are the physicians in the long term care industry that direct, coordinate, implement, and evaluate all spheres of professional services provided to clients in a nursing home setting. A medical director position includes both medical and administrative oversight of administrators, director of nurses, primary care providers, physician assistants, nurse practitioners, and physicians in training that practice in long term care facilities.

Medical direction provided by a medical director should combine both clinical knowledge and management capabilities in the physician's skill performance within the nursing home environment. A Medical Director must be a graduate from an accredited medical college with a degree in Internal Medicine/Family Practice, posses' liability insurance, and maintain a license that is in good standing with the state of issuance and practice.

In 1974, The Department of Health, Education and Welfare implemented strategies requiring all skilled nursing home facilities to retain a part-time or full-time Medical Director on staff. The 1987, OBRA (Ombudsman Reconciliation Act) passed regulatory guidelines requiring all long-term care facilities to staff a Medical Director for the following duties —

- Oversight of medical care provided to residents; providing clinical guidance.
- Reviewing and coordinating resident care policies and procedures that reflect current standards of practice.
- Implementing and demonstrating professional standards.
- Acquiring strategies for improvement and prevention of decline in quality care services.

A Medical Director should be allowed four to eight administrative hours per 100 beds in a facility to ensure adequate performed duties in a long-term care institution. The AMDA (American Medical Directors Association) recommends a pay base of 200-300 dollars per hour to be paid for the physician's services within the long-term care industry. Administrative functions in this position may also include attending quality assurance meetings, participating in surveys and inspections, coordinating plan of correction process, economic budgeting, employee health programs, assisting in obtaining consultants for a facility, utilization review, chart review, and educational processes with staff.

In the absence of any attending physician, with no replacement identified, a Medical Director will resume responsibility of the attending physician in the nursing home setting. A Medical Director will act as a facilities representative within the medical and social community; monitoring and educating primary care providers about long-term care structure as required in the healthcare profession.

Medical Directors must demonstrate leadership qualities and standards to motivate, inspire, and obtain results with direction provided within the long-term care industry. Distinguishing leadership character standards that are preferred in the long-term care industry include, but are not limited to the following —

- Demonstrate by example, assisting as needed the Administrator and Director of Nursing in accordance with goals of the department/corporation.
- Encourage team member development.
- Formulate solutions that promote building blocks in the team.
- Give positive feedback when deserved.

Effective Communication:

- Demonstrate respectful communication patterns, verbal and written.
- Be consistent with directives provided.
- Listen effectively and respond appropriately.
- Keep all lines of communication open — direct line staff to senior level management.

Ethical and Moral Character:

- Demonstrate behaviors that are in accordance with high moral standing.
- Be honest and truthful in all interactions.
- Set the standard for appropriate behaviors — hold staff to the same standard.

  Take accountability for mistakes.

  Treat all individuals the same (no favoritism).

  Demonstrate healthy psychological processes (no mind games).

  Allow autonomy and individuality as appropriate.

  Encourage kindness in relationship interactions.

Heighten Excellence:

- Allow staff to verbalize and instill improvement standards.
- Demonstrate and encourage high standard customer service.
- Attend Quality Assurance meetings and assist in implementing strategies to improve / sustain quality of care.
- Encourage communicative feedback with all staff.

Continuing Education:

- Encourage on-going educational processes with staff.
- Obtain own needed or required educational processes.
- Educate staff as desired or needed in the facility.

Develop and Maintain Trust:

- Be consistent with all forms of communication.
- Demonstrate follow through with actions, following verbalizations. (Actions and words are congruent)
- Allow time for questions by staff.

Demonstrate Respectful Mannerisms:

- Relationship interactions demonstrated with the mind set of equality.
- Encourage and practice relationship interactions that promote staff self-esteem.
- Develop and demonstrate psychological processes that promote psychological well-being in the work environment.

Empowerment:

- Give staff the opportunity and privilege to practice autonomy as allowed by scope of practice.
- Allow staff to learn and grow from minor mistakes.
- Acknowledge positive performance levels of staff.

Maintain Confidentiality:

- Keep all written and verbal communication concerning patients and staff within the facility.
- Do not discuss with colleagues any facility information.

A sense of humor is appreciated in the long-term care industry, well most of the time. The following story will add to the appreciation of physician's documentation (penmanship) within the healthcare continuum.

Patty: Receives orders from an orthopedic physician in the community in regards to a returning client, and states, "I can't read these orders. Can anyone else decipher what they say?"

The nurse proceeds to call the medical office for clarification of the physician's written orders.

Medical office nurse: Returns the phone call from Patty and clarifies the physician's written orders.

Two Weeks Later — The orthopedic physician phones the facility asking for nurse Patty.

Physician: "I can't read your request on the written telephone order. What is it that you want?"

Patty (who has perfect penmanship) exclaims, "What? You can't read what I wrote!"

Physician starts laughing.

Patty hangs up the phone and is upset over the physician's prank.

The remainder of nurses in the facility did find some humor in the joke, although under the strain of work, not everyone is relaxed enough to be able to respond as expected. It is these types of humorous dynamics that maintain structure and build relationships in the long-term care environment and medical community.

Medical Directors that perform in their positions effectively will support a corporations mission statement, as implemented by the corporation or private sector nursing facility, to assist in generating a shared vision for the staff; supporting the continuance of quality of healthcare delivery systems. The CMS (Centers for Medicare and Medicaid Services) instilled the F 501 tag "Medical Director" to be utilized in the survey process, and a facility to maintain federal regulatory compliance must —

Have a designated Medical Director that is a licensed physician. The physician must perform functions of a Medical Director position through —

a. The Medical Director providing input and assisting the facility to develop, review, and implement resident care policies based on current clinical standards.

b. The Medical Director assisting the facility in the coordination of medical care and services.

A Medical Director may also serve as an attending physician, but there is a difference in the two positions within the long-term care industry. The Medical Director is responsible for facility wide practices in the medical care encompassing nursing home structure.

A primary care provider or attending physician is responsible for the individual patient's medical care in a long-term care
environment.

Primary Care Providers

Attending physicians in the long-term care industry are required
to provide effective, efficient and appropriate medical services to all
clients that reside in nursing home facilities within the nation. Physicians play a very important role in the healthcare delivery systems
within communities and need to demonstrate excellence within the
medical continuum, including long-term care facilities.

Geriatrics in the long-term care setting involves a changing
group of clients ranging in differences with age, chronic disease
processes, cognitive abilities, functional abilities, culture, goals of
care provided, stay duration, death and dying processes, and acute
disease conditions or emergencies in nursing home facilities. Gerontological clients are a diverse population within the industry;
physicians need to acquire and maintain medical flexibility concerning their intellectual processes to generate and sustain high
level consultation, diagnosis, and treatment of clients in nursing
home settings. The focus in long-term care is different from acute
care, and physicians are required to shift their intellectual processes
to a mindset encompassing —

> Restoring and maintaining functional abilities
> Quality of life
> Comfort and dignity during the dying process
> Managing chronic disease processes
> Preventing and handling acute illnesses

Primary care physicians may delegate their responsibilities to
mid-level practitioners (physician assistants & nurse practitioners)
in the industry, insuring that mandatory requirements are met with
their patient obligations in long-term care facilities. All clinicians
that practice in the industry need to be knowledgeable about state
and federal regulatory guidelines managing long-term care facilities
in the nation to assist with regulatory compliance. Attending physician's duties include, but are not limited to the following —

- Unless seen for a history and physical within five days of admission, visit within 72 hours of admission and complete H&P (sign orders within a timely manner).

- Visit one time every 30 days for the first 90 days of stay.

- Visit every 60 days thereafter.

- Provide all orders including goals, advanced directives, medical diagnosis, substantiating diagnosis for medications, allergies, rehabilitative services, treatments, medications, labs, consultations, potential for discharge etc...

- Address all change in condition processes as notified i.e. falls, weight loss, pressure ulcers, weight gain, skin tears, acute illnesses, exacerbation of chronic illnesses, dying and death, hydration etc....

- Follow ethical standards set by the American Medical Association.

- Possess knowledge of Residents Rights.

Attending physicians are responsible for reporting to the Medical Director any concerns evolving in their practice within a nursing home facility. Primary care providers must demonstrate respectful relationship interactions to facilitate a positive work environment within the long-term care industry through professional maturity, team centered mentality, practicing confidentiality, and maintaining flexibility in mental processes about viewpoints and diversity of other individuals in nursing home environments. Physicians are required to work with facility staff and medical staff to sustain high quality proactive services delivered to clients and to maintain cost effective clinical standards within the nursing home setting.

The following physician scenario will assist individuals to understand the diversity of patients in the industry and the patience levels of physicians that serve their needs in the long-term care environment.

Mary's story

Mary was an elderly woman diagnosed with schizophrenia. She had been admitted to a nursing home after the Neurogeriatric Center she resided in had closed. The dynamics evolved as follows —

Mary: "Doctor, Doctor, There is something on my butt. I need you to get off whatever is on my butt."

Physician: "Oh, okay, let's go back to your room and take a look."

Mary: Runs back to her room stating, "I can feel it. There is something on my butt." Goes into her room, pulls down her pants, and lies down on the bed.

Physician: Examines the patient's bottom and sees a small amount of toilet tissue stuck to the resident's buttocks and states, "Oh, yes, I see. We will remove the substance from your bottom and you will be fine." Maintaining a professional demeanor during the process, the physician smiled and politely removed the toilet tissue from the client's buttocks.

Mary: "Thank you Doctor, that is so much better."

Attending physicians must possess more than patience and good humor, of course; they need a valid license to practice medicine that is in good standing within their state of practice. Primary care providers must also maintain a Drug Enforcement Administration (DEA) number and apply for medical staff membership in some nursing home facilities. Physicians must provide services within the long-term care industry in a professional manner consistent with standards governing their services; and in accordance with bylaws, rules, and regulations governing nursing home facilities. Effective and efficient skills are required in the primary care providers practice, due to a multidisciplinary approach of medical healthcare in nursing homes including —

Strong Analytical Skills   *Strong Diagnostic Skills*
Effective Communication Skills   *Strong Group Dynamic Skills*
Strong Problem Identification and Solving Skills

Primary care providers do affect quality of care services provided in the long-term care industry and are very important components surrounding quality assurance processes. Physicians that are efficient in their performance capabilities demonstrate thorough documentation, effective treatments and diagnostic tests ordered, obtain positive peer review results, and these physicians efforts improve state survey process results within the healthcare continuum in the long-term care industry.

Eden Alternative

Dr. William H. Thomas developed The Eden Alternative® philosophy in 1991, embarking on a process to deinstitutionalize nursing homes; through generating a home like atmosphere and environment for the elderly in the nation. The Eden philosophy views the aging process as a continuation of the quality of life; not death.

Dr. Thomas is a graduate of Harvard Medical School and a Board Certified Geriatrician, although he left full time medical practice in 2004. The Eden Alternative® non-profit organization was formally founded in 1994, and has grown to include facilities in other nations, plus all fifty states. Moving forward with his vision, Dr. Thomas also initiated The Green House® Project that was awarded a five year, ten million dollar grant in 2005 by the Robert Wood Johnson Foundation. The Green House® Project aims to tear down nursing homes in the nation and rebuild facilities into a home-like structure, assisting with the Eden philosophy.

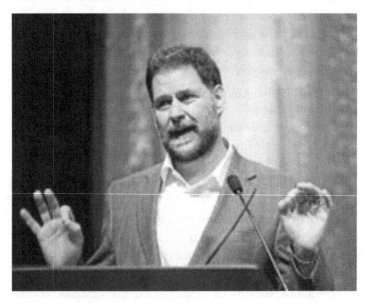

Dr. William Thomas "The Eden Alternative®."

There are around 300 nursing homes in the nation that practice The Eden Alternative® philosophy; these facilities report a reduction of infection rates, behavioral incidents, pressure ulcers, restraints, staff absenteeism, staff turnover, mortality rates, employee injuries, and overall number of prescription drugs within their facilities. A vision to eliminate loneliness, boredom, and helplessness based on a philosophy that the aging process should be a continuum of development and growth in life appears to decrease depression with the elderly client; thus facilitating many other positive outcomes from implementation of The Eden Alternative® in nursing home facilities. The Eden Alternative® has ten principles—

1. The three plagues of loneliness, helplessness and boredom account for the bulk of suffering among our elders.

2. An elder-centered community commits to creating a human habitat where life revolves around close and continuing contact with plants, animals, and children. It is these relationships that provide the young and old alike with a pathway to a life worth living.

3. Loving companionship is the antidote to loneliness. Elders deserve every access to human and animal companionship.

4. An elder-centered community creates opportunity to give as well as receive care. This is the antidote to helplessness.

5. An elder-centered community imbues daily life with variety and spontaneity by creating an environment in which unexpected and unpredictable interactions and happenings can take place. This is the antidote to boredom.

6. Meaningless activity corrodes the human spirit. The opportunity to do things that we find meaningful is essential to human health.

7. Medical treatment should be the servant of genuine human caring, never its master.

8. An elder-centered community honors its elders by de-emphasizing top-down bureaucratic authority, seeking instead to replace the maximum possible decision-making authority into the hands of the elders or into the hands of those closest to them.

9. Creating an elder-centered community is a never-ending process. Human growth must never be separated from human life.

10. Wise leadership is the lifeblood of any struggle against the three plagues. For it there can be no substitute.

Harry's story

Harry's situation demonstrates the down-to-earth mentality required at times in long-term care and that nursing home environments can be utilized as a stepping stone for healing within the healthcare continuum.

Harry was admitted to the long-term care facility after his hospitalization, due to a fractured clavicle and hip sustained from a fall at home. Harry had been receiving rehabilitative services encompassing physical and occupational therapy for approximately two weeks in the nursing home environment.

Harry: "Doc, When can I go home? I don't sleep well here. I want to go home."

Physician: "Well, Harry. Are you going to the bathroom by yourself yet?"

Harry: Looks down. "No."

Physician: "How can you go home if you can't use the bathroom alone yet?"

Harry: "I can figure out a way to do it."

The physician is very practical and down to earth with her response.

Physician: "I tell you what. You have to be able to wipe your own butt before you can go home. When I come in here and you can wipe your own butt, you can go home. Okay."

Utilizing The Eden Alternative® philosophy through creating long-term care facilities that foster a home like environment with gardens, plants, cats, dogs, birds, children, social networking, fish, functional activities, mutual respect and companionship, open dining schedules, buffet meals allowing selection, and generating autonomy in services received and delivered in nursing home structure assists the elderly client through the aging process. This philosophy enables our elderly in the nation to evolve through the aging process in a healthier manner. The Eden philosophy maintains self-esteem and self-worth in the human spirit with clients assisting in sustaining psychological and physical health encompassing clients in the nursing home environment.

Some states have developed Grant Assistance Programs to assist long-term care industry facilities with the progression of change concerning this philosophy in nursing homes. In one state, grant money was generated from a Nursing Home Resident Trust Account established from State civil monetary penalties, collected through enforcement activities against nursing homes; the funds were utilized to assist in instilling the Eden philosophy process in long-term care structures within their state.

In any case, improving the quality of life for the elderly is a very positive contribution for any person or institution to make. We owe a deep felt thank-you to Dr. Thomas for perceiving this requirement for improving the care provided to the older population. It is the vision and intellectual processes of individuals like Dr. Thomas that assist in continuous evolution and progression of gerontological care, addressing a holistic model of physical, psychological, spiritual, and psychosocial well-being of all human beings within nursing home facilities.

Quality Indicator Survey

Dr. Andrew Kramer attended Harvard Medical School and is responsible for developing and implementing the Quality Indicator Survey process, which he initiated in 1993 at the University of Colorado. The Centers for Medicare and Medicaid Services has contracted with Dr. Kramer to initiate a nationwide establishment of the Quality Indicator Survey process; and Dr. Kramer is responsible for the education and training operations surrounding this survey process in the United States. Dr. Kramer has over 26 years of experience in medical / health care research and research management. Research performed by Dr. Kramer focuses on the quality of care in long-term care facilities, rehabilitation hospitals, and home health agencies in the nation.

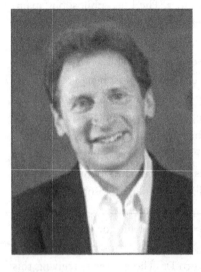

Dr. Andrew Kramer

"Quality Indicator Survey"

The Quality Indicator Survey will be replacing the Traditional Standard Survey process conducted annually in nursing homes throughout the nation as all state surveyors are trained in this process. Dr. Kramer is the Director of the Center for Health Services Research at the University of Colorado and directs the implementation, training, support and refinement of current QIS processes being initiated by CMS in the United States.

It is believed that this survey process will be more accurate in identifying care dynamics within long-term care facilities, thus assisting in improving the quality of care for elderly clients in our nation. Dr. Kramer must be acknowledged and appreciated for his research contribution that will assist in continuous quality improvement strategies within the long-term care industry. This process supports psychological processes of quality assurance and quality of care improvement for the geriatric population within the nation through research programs that generate proactive change in survey processes within nursing homes.

Focus

Physicians in all positions within the gerontological profession contribute to standards of care provided in the industry. It is their contribution of medical knowledge base, ethical standards, quality assurance and quality improvement models that assist in the evolvement of continuous improvement of quality of care and life for elderly clients within the nation. All physicians in the medical field that have contact with nursing homes do have a requirement for the knowledge base of state and federal regulatory guidelines monitoring the industry. Acute care settings in hospitals are not regulated by these guidelines, thus some physicians may not possess a requirement needed to understand why medical staff in long-term care perform procedures with certain modules not practiced in acute care settings within hospitals.

Continuous quality practices through effective communication will assist in decreasing the gap between acute care and long-term care services rendered in the medical arena; assisting in the transition processes for gerontological clients as they move between the two entities during their healthcare stays. Hopefully, improving and sustaining quality assurance and improvement standards in hospital and long-term care based industries.

Chapter Six. Interdisciplinary Team

An interdisciplinary team approach with services delivered is required in the healthcare and long-term care industry to meet both intrinsic and extrinsic needs of clients. The multidisciplinary team philosophy encompasses all the positions previously discussed and the following departments —

- Business Office Manager & Staff
- Activities Director & Staff
- Environmental Services Coordinator & Staff
- Social Services Manager & Staff
- Maintenance Supervisor & Staff
- Medical Records Coordinator & Staff
- Dietary Manager & Staff

Interdisciplinary team approaches also encompass external entities that provide services and consultation in specialty areas such as hospice, pharmaceuticals, rehabilitation, religion, surveys and educational processes. Providing quality care to clients is a multidisciplinary process and responsibility within the healthcare industry, and all individuals involved should possess a mindset surrounding a proactive preventative bases to accomplish goals related to improvement and maintenance of quality delivery of care services to clients in the nursing home environment. The following positions and departments discussed do indeed assist in providing a high level quality of services within long-term care and should be viewed as an important aspect involved with customer satisfaction in the nursing home environment.

Dietary Manager

A Certified Dietary Manager is responsible for the overall operation of the dietary department. This position ensures food quality for clients through directing and assisting in the preparation and serving of regular and therapeutic diets, ordering food and supplies for a facility, maintaining sanitary conditions with infection control strategies utilized, and ensuring a smooth operation of the dietary department in nursing home structure.

A dietary manager in the long-term care industry must be a graduate of a dietary manager's course that meets state and federal regulatory guidelines and must be certified by the Dietary Manager Association. Major responsibilities are to ensure that all safety and sanitation standards are above levels that are acceptable according to state and federal regulatory guidelines. Job responsibilities in this department include, but are not limited to—

- Directing and supervising dietary function and personnel (hires, orients, trains, counsels, disciplines and terminates employees).
- Maintaining budgetary guidelines of the department (cost records maintained).
- Scheduling employee hours.
- Checking in and maintaining inventories of food and supplies.
- Purchasing, producing and maintaining a timely service of food.
- Completing initial dietary assessment and screening of clients (records food preferences and allergies).
- Processing new diet orders and diet changes; checks with physician orders (keeps diet cards updated).
- Visiting clients one time per quarter and completing monthly dietary notes.
- Working effectively with dietician consultant to ensure quality nutritious meals are served in the nursing home.

- Maintaining current care plan for each client.
- Completing MDS sections and participating in care plan meetings.
- Attending Quality Assurance meetings, assisting Director of Nursing with monitoring weight loss and weight gain dynamics according to regulatory guidelines.
- Inspecting storage areas weekly for temperature and cleanliness.

Dietary managers perform the initial dietary consultation, and assessment processes can evolve into an interesting scenario with some clients in nursing home structure. A petite female client in one nursing home was particularly specific in her food consumption and choices. Deloris's situation evolved as follows —

Deloris's story

Deloris was admitted to the nursing home after her husband passed away and she was no longer able to care for herself in her residence.

Dietary Manager: *"Hello, Deloris. My name is Jane. I need to perform an assessment to meet your nutritional needs and desires while you stay with us. Is this a good time?"*

Deloris: *"Yes, I suppose we can discuss this now. I am very particular about my diet and I want to be sure you prepare it correctly."*

Dietary Manager: *"OK. Let's get started. Do you have any food allergies?"*

Deloris: *"Oh yes."* And initiates a long list of food samples. *"I am allergic to shellfish, milk, pork, eggs, liver, spinach, artichokes, carrots, broccoli, tuna, orange juice etc......"*

Dietary Manager: *"Are these all foods you are allergic to, or do you just not like them?"*

Deloris: *"Well, I guess I don't like some of them, but I don't want them served to me, so I am allergic."*

The dietary manager smiled and simply complied with Deloris's requests. . Demonstrating the requirement for conforming to and maintaining residents rights in the long-term care facility; dietary managers will set an example for structuring a psychology of practicing by mandated state / federal regulated guidelines.

Medical Records Coordinator

Medical Records Managers are responsible for planning, developing, and administering health information systems that comply with standards of state and federal regulatory guidelines in long-term care facilities. Both, paper and computerized based medical record information are utilized in the long-term care industry and management skills in both record keeping strategies are required to sustain proficiency concerning medical information data bases. A medical records manager will assist in the privacy, safety, and security of all health information within a nursing home setting. Additional duties in this position can include —

- Implementing departmental policies and procedures.
- Overseeing the departmental budget.
- Participating in Quality Assurance meetings.
- Following HIPPA guidelines and providing guidance to staff.
- Ensuring all charts are in proper order including mandated regulatory information.
- Evaluating and stripping charts when required.
- Following policies and procedures with all health information that leaves and enters a facility.

Most medical records coordinators in nursing home settings have a Bachelor's Degree in health information management or a related healthcare or technology field. It is required by some entities that an individual must also possess the RHIA; Registered Health Information Administrator's certification. Medical records managers will direct staff in the areas of coding, transcription, release of information and medical record filing in long-term care structure.

Activities Director

The Activities Director position requires an individual to plan, develop, organize and implement a system of ongoing activities in the nursing home setting that meets regulatory requirements;

providing physical, psychological, and psychosocial well-being for long-term care clients through various activity stimulation series. Educational basis for an activities director consists of at least a high school diploma and completion of a state approved activities director training program. This position could also be occupied by a qualified recreation therapist, activities professional certified, occupational therapist, or occupational therapist assistant within the long-term care industry.

A developed activity program system should provide activities for clients on a daily basis, including evenings and weekends. Activities need to be appropriate; meeting the requirements of nursing home clients, based from the activities comprehensive assessment and could include—

Group social activities	*Religious based programs*
One to one activities	*Exercise programs*
Board games or card games	*Educational systems*
Indoor and outdoor programs	
Activities outside of a facility	
Hobbies such as: arts, crafts, plays, reading,	

Activity directors need to develop support systems within nursing home settings and communities to assist in the program functional abilities; through networking with clients and family systems. Interpersonal skills and patience are necessary personality traits for this position, due to working with individuals of varying developmental, psychological, intellectual, and physical functional levels. The activities director must also possess an ability to motivate others; encouraging participation in activities delivered to clients in the long-term care industry.

Activity directors are required to spend at least thirty minutes of staff time per resident per week in activity related services. It is also federally regulated that the activities calendar be posted in large print within an area accessible to all clients within a nursing home environment. There are other management and duty requirements with an activity director position that could encompass—

- Supervising activity assistant directors or activity aides.
- Recruiting, training, and supervising volunteers.

- Documenting MDS sections, progress notes, and care plan strategies (including goals).
- Completing comprehensive activity assessments.
- Procuring necessary equipment and supplies.
- Participating in departmental budget development.
- Attending care plan, quality assurance, behavior management committee, weight management committee, and department head meetings.

An activities assistant director assists the activities director with providing an activity program that meets client's needs in the nursing home environment. The goal is accomplished through assessment of resident functional abilities, preferences in activities, planning for and providing group / individualized activities, and meeting regulatory requirements within the department.

Educational requirements for an assistant director must be a high school diploma level or completion of a state approved activities director course. The activities assistant director will assist with both group and individualized activities in the long-term care environment. Assigned duties for an assistant are designated by the activities director and could include: setting up the activity area, assisting with transportation, observing participation and responses, documentation on activities records, interacting appropriately, and having awareness of individual clients needs and responding to those needs during interaction processes. An assistant director will assume responsibility of the activities department in the absence of the activities director within the long-term care industry.

Activities programming is a very important aspect of the nursing home environment to some clients as demonstrated below —

Fern's story

Fern: "Are we playing Bingo today?"

Activities Director: "No, not today, Fern. Bingo is on Wednesday afternoons."

Fern: "What day is today?"

Activities Director: "Today is Monday."

Fern: "Well, we need to increase the number of days for Bingo. I like Bingo, and I want to play it every day."

Activities Director: "Fern, I don't think we can set up Bingo for every day, but I'll see what I can do for volunteers to increase the number of days per week."

Fern: "Really?"

Activities Director: "Yes, really."

The Activities Director was able to enlist the assistance of several volunteers from the community to increase bingo to Monday, Wednesday and Friday afternoons, thus meeting Fern's and other clients' psychosocial needs through increasing socialization processes in the nursing home environment.

An activity aide or assistant assists the activities director in deliverance of the activity program as directed by the activities director in a nursing home. An individual in this position must possess at least a high school diploma. Activity aides could assist in both group and individualized activities including: delivering and reading mail, 1:1 interactions, promoting participation in activity programs, assisting in chaperoning activities off facility grounds, transportation to and from activities, and monitoring client requirements during activity sessions. Duties for an activity aide could also include assisting with deliverance of monthly activity calendars, filing photographs, and keeping closet storage areas organized. Activity aides will keep an activity program functioning in the absence of the activities director within a facility.

Social Services Manager

A Social Services Manager in the long-term care industry plays a major role in enabling each individual client to function at their highest level possible of social and emotional wellness. Social workers offer guidance and counseling to individuals through specific casework, group work, and community organization work. Most corporations and long-term care facilities require individuals in this position to have a Master's Degree in social work, but there are some positions and institutions that will accept a Bachelor's Degree in the required specialty field.

Individuals in social workers positions usually major in sociology, psychology, or another social science. Courses encompassing this degree include economics, political science, human growth and development, methods of social work, and general education classes. The National Association of Social Workers may certify individuals after two years of supervised work; enhancing eligibility into the Academy of Certified Social Workers. Social services managers and social workers in the long-term care industry have many responsibilities and some may include —

Assisting in client admission and discharge processes:
Pre-admit Screening
Advance Directives
Power of Attorney (financial & healthcare)
Social History
Marketing and touring of facilities.

Psychosocial assessments:
MDS Section
Care Planning
Documentation in progress notes

Counseling clients & families:
Crisis intervention
Problem solving
Complaint resolution
Problem identification
Ensuring social & emotional needs of clients are met.
Promoting maximum levels of client independence.
Advocating & protecting resident's rights.
Educating clients and staff.
Contacting and recruiting community resources.
Ensuring financial assistance needs are met of clients.
Enlisting the assistance of volunteers.
Promoting social contact and interaction within a facility.

Environmental Services Coordinator

The Environmental Services Coordinator manages the housekeeping and laundry services within a long-term care facility; ensuring a clean, safe, odor free, and orderly environment. Individuals in this position plan, develop, direct, supervise and implement services provided by housekeeping and laundry staff maintaining sanitary and infection control processes through delivered professional duties in the industry. Educational requirements are that the individual has a high school diploma, and four to five years of housekeeping experience, preferably in a long-term care environment.

Management duties in this position include hiring, training and terminating employees; assigning personnel to designated work regions; scheduling staff hours; assisting with budget development and maintenance; inspecting work regions for compliance of regulatory guidelines; assessing client satisfaction with services rendered; implementing proactive preventative strategies to promote safety; and assisting in policy and procedure development for the departments. Duties also designated to this position could include —

- Purchasing of cleaning supplies, chemicals, paper products and departmental equipment.
- Maintaining inventory levels.
- Ensuring all departments receive supplies as needed to function effectively.
- Obtaining cost estimates from department capital purchases.
- Ensuring Health Department regulations and Fire Marshall regulations are met.

Ensuring all clients personal clothing is appropriately cared for in the long-term care environment can be a challenge at times, some family systems elect to perform their own loved one's services and others prefer the facility to provide laundry services. Harold's case displays the need to use effective written and verbal communication within nursing home facilities.

Harold's story

Harold was admitted to the long-term care facility after a recent cerebral vascular accident and during the admission process his family elected to provide laundry services for Harold during his nursing home stay.

Nursing Staff: "We need to send all of Harold's personal clothing to laundry to be labeled and then it will be returned to his room."

Family: "That is fine. As long as the clothing is returned to the room for my wife to pick it up once a week for laundering."

Nursing Staff: "Yes Sir, we will ensure everyone knows the family prefers to provide Harold's laundry services."

A week passes and the family visits the facility to pick up Harold's laundry. The personal clothing items had been labeled and returned to the client's room, yet there was no laundry waiting in the personal laundry basket in the private room. Speaking to a charge nurse, the following conversation evolved between staff and family members —

Family: "We asked to do Harold's laundry and yet no clothing is in his basket."

Charge Nurse: "Let me look into the situation."

Family: "Please do; we do not want the facility providing laundry services for our father."

Nurse: After evaluating the situation. "Apparently, there was a break in the communication pattern of your request. I sent a request slip to laundry services and I will place a sign up in Harold's room to ensure all staff are aware of your request to provide laundry services for Harold. This should stop personal clothing items from being sent to the laundry department. I am so sorry that the lines of communication were broken and we did not follow through with your request on admission."

Family: "As long as we get the issue resolved, I do not see a problem."

As the manager of laundry services, an individual needs to maintain quality and timely delivery of laundry to clients in the nursing home setting. Laundry managers also need to inspect work environments frequently to ensure clean, sanitary linens and personal clothes are delivered to appropriate entities within the long-term care industry.

Laundry aides under the direction of the environmental services coordinator will perform duties of collection, processing, distribution and inventory of linens and personal clothing consistent with facility policy and procedures and regulatory guidelines. Duties for laundry aides may include, but are not limited to —

- Weighing and sorting linens for processing
- Operating irons, folders, and presses as required
- Folding and sorting personal clothing and institutional linens
- Auditing linens for required labels and repairs
- Delivering personal and institutional linens to units
- Discarding unusable linens and records
- Reporting equipment malfunction
- Ensuring economical utilization of products

Maintenance Supervisor

Maintenance Supervisors in the long-term care industry coordinate maintenance departments to ensure a safe environmental living area for clients. An individual in this position is responsible for preventative maintenance and maintenance of: air conditioning units, refrigeration, plumbing, electrical, and communication systems. Waste disposal, snow removal and pest control are also included in the job requirements for a maintenance supervisor in nursing home facilities.

Educational requirements for maintenance supervisors are at least a high school degree and five years of experience as a maintenance worker. An associate's degree or a higher degree level in building maintenance is preferred in most institutions, sustaining coursework and knowledge base concerning blueprint reading; facility maintenance; budget planning; accounting; management principles; building codes; and electrical, heating and plumbing systems. Knowledge base of OSHA (Occupational Safety Health Administration) standards and Life Safety Codes are mandatory; ensuring that smoke detectors, heat detectors, and fire alarm systems work effectively and efficiently in all nursing home facilities within the nation.

State licensure is usually not required for a maintenance supervisor, except in cases where they actually perform electrical and plumbing procedures. Certification can be obtained through the International Management Institute (IMI) and consists of the Certified Maintenance Professional (CMP) for individuals with a high school degree and Certified Maintenance Manager (CMM) for those individuals with an associate's degree or higher level of education. Other duties in this position encompass —

- Routinely inspecting buildings to identify maintenance problems.
- Creating work assignments for staff.
- Hiring, training, promoting, supervising and terminating employees.
- Completing performance evaluations.
- Generating work schedules.
- Planning & implementation of departmental budgets.
- Maintaining inventory.
- Coordination of remodeling or redecorating projects.
- Supervising delivery of freight.

Business Office Manager

The long-term care industry utilizes Business Office Managers to generate and sustain effective financial functions for facilities. Individuals in this position are required to possess at least an associate's degree in business administration or management.

Knowledge base of Medicare, Medicaid, and Managed Care insurance billing is mandatory for this position. Most businesses require an individual employed as a business office manager to have at least three years of experience in third party billing and collections to obtain employment concerning this position in the nursing home industry. Typical duties in this position are —

- Managing payroll.
- Ordering office supplies.
- Planning travel.
- Monitoring billing and collection activities.
- Assuring proper accounting procedures and controls are utilized.
- Analyzing collections on a monthly basis.
- Ensuring an accurate and timely closing at month end.

- Maintaining records and submitting records accurately and timely according to state and federal regulatory guidelines.
- Maintaining employee files.
- Processing data and maintaining security.

A degree in Business Administration elicits skill sets in records and information management, personnel management, facility maintenance and management, office administration, and business communication. Obtaining a Certified Manager Designation from the Institute of Certified Professional Managers (CPM) will assist in credibility as a professional in a business office manager position within the long-term care industry.

Quality Assurance Strategies

Managers in the long-term care industry utilize two different philosophies with services delivered; (QA) quality assurance and (CQI) continuous quality improvement. Both philosophies assist with business delivery systems, but differ slightly in their approach and vision. Quality assurance processes deter, identify, and correct issues associated with services rendered that do not meet standards of quality performance. Quality improvement processes seek to continuously enhance services delivered through evaluating and modifying systems in place within a facility.

Nursing home managers utilize both intrinsic and extrinsic systems to improve and sustain services within the long-term care industry. Intrinsic systems are processes such as mock surveys; weekly tracking meetings; monthly assurance meetings; daily rounds; daily charting logs; monthly chart audits; and monthly consultations performed by: nurse consultants, pharmacists, dieticians, and rehabilitation staff. Extrinsic system processes include yearly state health inspection surveys, yearly safety code inspection surveys, OSHA surveys, and complaint surveys.

Both intrinsic and extrinsic systems if utilized effectively will assist in effective monitoring of quality of services provided in the long-term care industry; improving and sustaining quality of care for the elderly in our nation. For the purpose of current discussion we will focus more on the intrinsic systems utilized in the nursing home setting.

Intrinsic quality assurance or improvement strategies are formulated, implemented, monitored, and evaluated by middle management personnel in the long-term care arena. Monthly quality assurance meetings require the administrator, the medical director and all department heads to be present, assisting in monitoring compliance with federal regulatory guidelines. Each department head is required to verbally and in written form identify problems or potential problems within their department, and present resolutions for improvement during the quality assurance meetings. Follow through is maintained through secretarial documentation of meeting minutes notes recorded and being reviewed each subsequent meeting, until sufficient resolution is obtained and sustained within the specific departments.

Weekly meetings that should be performed in the nursing department to monitor data are:

- Weight loss/gain committee meetings
- Psychotropic medication/behavior committee meetings
- Pressure ulcer/skin committee meetings
- Fall/accident/restraints committee meetings
- Medicare/rehabilitation committee meetings

During the specified nursing meetings, data is evaluated regarding identified areas of concern with proactive preventative interventions assessed, reevaluated and implemented as required to decrease potential problems or the continuation of current problems. This process assists in improving quality of healthcare delivery systems in the nursing home environment. Quality care indicators need to be monitored on a weekly to monthly basis as formulated from the MDS (minimum data set) in specified meetings to assure continuous quality improvement strategies are effective as implemented through evaluation of statistical data surrounding falls, weight loss, pressure ulcers, restraints, infection control processes etc..; within the long-term care industry.

Daily rounds performed by all department heads to assess, monitor, evaluate, supervise and educate as required to maintain compliance with strategies implemented assists in improving quality of services delivered. The daily rounds also assist with maintaining quality assurance philosophies and strategies each supervisor is responsible for in their specific department and correcting procedural deficiencies if identified in nursing home structure within a facility.

Nurse Consultants conduct monthly audits of all departments in corporate owned nursing home facilities. This process assists in identifying potential deficient areas within the long-term care industry. Mock surveys are also performed by nurse consultants as the time period for annual state survey inspection nears, assisting in identifying potential deficient areas prior to a state survey process. Typically, long-term care facilities have a 90 day window from the date of the last health inspection to the present inspection process, thus a consultant can approximate the time period of conduction of a subsequent survey; assisting in correcting any identified problematic areas in a facility prior to the actual regulated survey inspection.

Dietician and pharmacist consultants visit long-term care facilities on a monthly basis; performing chart, record, and procedural audits. These two entities monitor their areas of expertise to ensure regulatory guidelines are being practiced in regards to pharmacy and dietary standards of practice. The dietary manager and director of nursing are responsible for assisting consultants while present in a facility; notifying consultants of current issues identified within their departments; promoting continuous quality improvement processes in nursing home environments within the nation.

Focus

It is easy to identify that an interdisciplinary team is a necessity in the long-term care industry. A multitude of potential prospective dynamics or situations that can evolve require many professionals and several implemented systems to provide continuous quality improvement services to the elderly within the nursing home environment. Interdisciplinary teams that place their focus on proactive preventative interventions do succeed in decreasing quality indicator data; thus improving quality of care delivery systems for the elderly client in nursing homes within the nation. Assistance of

extrinsic quality assurance strategies add to the success of intrinsic continuous quality improvement systems; obtaining a desired
outcome of above standard quality of care delivery systems for the
elderly in the United States.

CHAPTER SEVEN. SURVEY PROCESSES

Extrinsic quality assurance strategies encompass various survey processes in the long-term care industry. Survey processes ensure federal and state regulatory guidelines are being implemented and followed in the nursing home setting within the nation, assisting in meeting quality of care standards for elderly clients within the medical profession. Through various survey processes an institution can be inspected more than once during a year's time, maintaining quality of care services rendered in a facility; even in cases surrounding problematic nursing homes. Mandatory yearly survey processes for all nursing homes consists of the—

Health and Human Services Survey
Life Safety Code Survey

Additional survey processes may transpire or could be performed if requested by a nursing home administrator. An example would be the OSHA (Occupational Safety and Health Administration) survey. OSHA surveyors will inspect a nursing home upon request and provide recommendations for improvement based on their assessments in a long-term care facility. The Joint Commission (TJC), formerly known as Joint Commission on Accreditation of Healthcare Organizations (JCAHO) will survey long-term care facilities for accreditation if requested by specific facilities or corporations. Other survey processes that could transpire per request or unannounced are —

Federal Surveys   Complaint Surveys
Quality Indicator Surveys

It has been stated by some news media that long-term care facilities are actually regulated more strictly than nuclear power plants in the nation. This in and of itself is a very positive attribute for the elderly population in the United States. State and federal authorities regulating the quality of gerontological nursing, medical services, and living environments for the elderly in our nation demonstrates that as a nation we do respect our elders and work to enforce and maintain quality of care delivery systems in nursing home environments.

Traditional Health Inspection

Nurse health inspection state surveyors are mandated to be a registered nurse with a Bachelor's or Master's Degree and to possess a current licensure in the state of practice. It is preferred that a nurse employed in a state surveyor position provide an employment history of at least three years of long-term care experience. Registered nurses in these positions also have to complete a CMS (Centers for Medicare and Medicaid Services) long-term care federal basic training course in HCFA headquarters and successfully complete the Survey Minimum Qualifications test. A state surveyor of long-term care facilities must possess basic knowledge, skills and competencies surrounding areas of —

Medical facilities   Survey tasks & protocols
Long-term care facilities   MDS training programs
Inspection   Nurse aide training programs
Investigation   Gerontological nursing
Regulatory methods   Licensed dietetics
Medical terminology   Social work
Coding
Principles & operation of healthcare administration
Federal & state regulations

The primary job purpose for a health care facility surveyor is to perform onsite inspections and / or surveys of services rendered, or care providers and suppliers to determine compliance with Medicare and Medicaid program participation requirements and state licensure laws. Each surveyor's role on a survey team is based on their level of expertise and assigned discipline: nurse, dietician, or social worker experience levels and educational knowledge base.

All nursing home facilities must be in compliance with federally mandated requirements to maintain payment systems from Medicare and Medicaid institutions. At the minimum a standard health inspection and life safety code survey needs to be conducted annually within each long-term care institution in the nation. Surveys / inspections are conducted at least within a fifteen month interval between each inspection; with an average of an every twelve month cycle occurring in most states within the United States.

A survey team size will vary depending on the size and census of each nursing home inspected. Also taken into consideration determining team size are known past complaints and deficiencies cited within a facility. Members of the team may vary: all nursing home standard survey processes must have at least one registered nurse on the survey team.

Social workers, registered dieticians, pharmacists, activity professionals, and rehabilitative specialists will be implemented on survey teams, when possible or applicable within the survey processes in the nation.

The length of a survey will vary from institution to institution based on the size of a facility and / or complexity of issues identified as problems or possible problems within the nursing home. All nursing home surveys are conducted unannounced; maintaining an ability to observe and review care practices that are typical for each facility. At least ten percent of all standard health inspection surveys must be conducted on off hours including: weekends, holidays, and before 8 AM or after 6 PM with consecutive days utilized during the survey process. The following types of institutions within the healthcare arena will be surveyed and certified annually in the medical profession —

- State operated skilled nursing facilities
- State operated nursing facilities
- State operated dual facilities

- Non-state operated nursing facilities
- Non-state operated dual facilities (skilled facilities/non-skilled facilities)

The survey process initiates for surveyors prior to entering a facility through evaluating the institutions quality indicators based from MDS data, past deficiencies, personnel changes, and Ombudsman information. OSCAR (online survey certification and reporting system) reports are utilized to obtain data about previous survey results, number of certified beds, address of the facility etc...; prior to the actual in-house survey of a nursing home.

State surveyors use three regulation sets to assess quality of care delivery systems: Federal long-term care regulations / state operations manual, state minimum licensing requirements, and the state standards for payment requirements in accordance with each states specific standards.

When a survey team enters a facility they will identify themselves and hold an entrance conference. Survey team members have a specific process that they progress through to assist them in identifying compliance with regulatory guidelines in long-term care facilities. The process initially begins with a tour of the facility conducted by the Director of Nursing and / or Administrator. After the tour, survey team members will assess data obtained prior to the facility entrance and evaluate client's records to pick their resident sample for evaluation during the survey process.

The number of clients in their sample is based on the census (number of clients in the facility) at the time of the survey and occurs in two stages. In stage one, sixty percent of the clients in the sample are picked based on off-site preparation information and data, and tour of the facility. In stage two, the other forty percent of the sample clients are identified from concerns observed or unresolved in stage one, including clients with pressure ulcers, weight loss, dehydration, falls, infections, decline in status etc.... It is federally regulated that the sample must include at least one client from each of the following categories: interviewable, minimal care clients; interviewable, maximum care clients; non-interviewable minimal care clients; and non-interviewable maximum care clients.

Surveyors will then conduct information gathering that encompasses the following —

- General observation of the facility: environmental factors affecting patient's life, health, and safety.
- Kitchen, food service observations: storage, preparation and service.
- Resident Review: Holistic assessment of sampled residents including closed record reviews and dining observation. Review of nursing services, physician services, rehabilitative services, dental services, infection control, and client behavior.
- Quality of life assessment: Individual interviews, group interviews, family interviews, and observation. Activities and resident dignity review and observation.
- Medication pass & Pharmacy services: Observation of medication pass, medication error detection methodology, pharmacist services, review of policies and procedures concerning medications, storage and handling of medications.
- Quality Assessment & Assurance Review: Evaluation of quality assurance and continuous quality improvement processes in a facility.
- Abuse prohibition review: Assessment for developed policies and procedures that prohibit abuse and address resident rights.

State surveyors at times do possess a sense of humor and can exhibit this quality during a survey process, as exhibited in the following scenario.

Surveyor Kevin: "You need to ensure that the issues I covered with you yesterday are resolved and systems are in place to prevent ongoing problems with clients."

Nurse Kathy: "Yes, I will make sure everything you asked is completed."

Surveyor Kevin: Laughing. "OK, I chewed your left buttock yesterday, now today I am going to chew your right, let's get started."

Nurse Kathy: Starts laughing. She knows the surveyor is attempting to lighten the mood during the survey process, since it is her first survey as a Director of Nursing.

Positive survey outcomes will consist of either the facility is in compliance with program requirements and no deficiencies will be cited; or the facility is in substandard compliance with no deficiency occurring that is more serious than potentially causing a minor negative impact on a resident. Cited deficiencies with state health inspections are identified as "F" tags. Scope and severity of "F" tag deficiencies are categorized as demonstrated in the diagram below —

Scope of Deficiency

Severity of Deficiency	Isolated	Pattern	Widespread
Immediate jeopardy to resident health or safety	J	K	L
Actual harm that is not immediate jeopardy	G	H	I
No actual harm with potential for more than minimal harm that is not immediate jeopardy	D	E	F
No actual harm with Potential for minimal harm	A	B	C

Negative survey outcomes require a plan of correction to be submitted to the state agency by the nursing home, including how the deficiency or deficiencies are going to be corrected facility wide in an institution. An acceptable plan of correction (POC) and evidence provided that it has been implemented with no serious complaints cited, will elicit a state response of "presumed compliance" with scope levels of deficiencies surrounding "D" and "F" and no substandard quality of care identified in a nursing home.

Deficiencies that are cited that cause actual harm or immediate jeopardy to client safety, compromising a patient's ability to maintain or reach their highest level of physical, mental, and psychosocial well-being are attached scope levels of "G" or "I"; and "F" tag deficiencies likely to cause serious injury, harm, impairment, or death are attached scope levels of "J" or "L." In these cases, state surveyors must conduct an onsite resurvey processes to determine compliance with program requirements in a nursing home setting.

Substandard quality of care is determined by "F" tag deficiencies that cause harm and occur widespread in a facility. Scope levels of "J", "L", "H", "I", and "F" are attached to these deficiencies. State survey agencies determine a nursing homes compliance with program requirements and submit their outcome data on a long-term care facility to HCFA and / or the state Medicaid agency. Negative outcome survey processes will have remedies instituted by HCFA or the state Medicaid agency and may include —

Category 1: Directed plan of correction, state monitoring and / or directed in-service training.

Category 2: Denial of payment for new admissions, denial of payment for all clients imposed by HCFA and / or Civil money penalties of $50.00 to $3000 per day or single instance monetary penalties of $1000 - $10,000.

Category 3: Temporary management, termination. Civil penalties of $3050–$10,000 per day for non-compliance and / or a $1000–$10,000 penalty per instance.

Penalties are mandated by federal statutes for non-compliant nursing homes. Denial of payment for new admissions must be imposed by the state when a facility is not in compliance within three months of being found out of compliance by a survey team. Plus, denial of payment and state monitoring must be imposed with three consecutive substandard survey results in a long-term care facility. Termination of the provider agreement will be initiated when a facility is not within compliance during a six month time frame of being found non-compliant with regulatory guidelines. A finding of substandard quality of care in a nursing home will be reported to the state Ombudsman and the state board responsible for licensing an administrator in the non-compliant long-term care facility.

Extended surveys or partial extended surveys will be initiated when the team identifies or suspects substandard quality of care in a facility. Expansion of a survey may be conducted if surveyors suspect substandard quality of care, but can neither prove nor refute the belief and must obtain additional data to determine results, which could then transpire into an extended or partial extended survey process.

Surveyors at the termination of an inspection will hold an exit conference to present survey findings to the nursing home staff. Deficiencies will be discussed at the exit conference, but scope and severity may be withheld until the final survey report is submitted. Additional information could be provided to surveyors by nursing home staff to refute deficiencies, if applicable during the exit conference.

When long-term care facility management personnel do not agree with a deficiency or the scope of a deficiency that constitutes substandard care, they have the option of requesting an IDR, Informal Dispute Resolution. The request should state the deficiencies being disputed and filed within the ten calendar day regulations governing the plan of correction. Nursing home facilities are allowed to utilize resources such as an attorney to assist with formulation of an IDR submission to the state. It is the state's responsibility to make decisions for non-compliance surrounding an Informal Dispute Resolution procedure and CMS holds the states accountable for their decision making processes in regards to the informal dispute resolution system.

Complaint surveys are conducted when customers file complaints with the state Health and Human Services Department or the state Ombudsman. These inspections are unannounced and can occur both off-site and on-site to gather data and information about an alleged complaint within a nursing home. Submitted complaints are logged according to severity of the allegation; immediate jeopardy cases are handled immediately and all other cases are assessed from seven to forty-five days from the date of filing. Complaint surveys concentrate on the specific area of concern and can initiate into an expanded or traditional survey. Surveyor's will make their decisions based on data obtained, and expand or upgrade the survey if warranted to gather more information. Conclusion of a complaint survey process will result in the allegation being substantiated or unsubstantiated, with reports submitted and consequential action initiated if required within a long-term care facility.

Life Safety Code Survey

The State Fire Marshall is responsible for conducting the Life Safety Code inspection in long-term care facilities. Deficiencies with the life safety code inspection are identified as "K: tags. During a life safety code inspection the fire marshal evaluates the facility's structure, preventative maintenance, fire control features and overall safety for clients residing in the facility. Some of the areas assessed consist of these—

- The facility must be constructed with non-combustible materials and building elements, including walls, columns, and floors.
- If the roof is constructed with combustible material it is protected by a properly installed and maintained wet-pipe automatic sprinkler system.
- The facility must be designed in accordance with national, regional, state or local building codes to provide protection from building collapse or failure of essential equipment from earthquake hazards, tornadoes, hurricanes, and other natural disasters.
- Roads, fire lanes, and parking areas must permit unrestricted access for emergency vehicles.
- The facility must ensure the roof membrane does not permit water to penetrate the roof.
- Compact shelving if utilized must be designed to permit proper air circulation and fire protection.
- The facility must have an integrated pest management program.
- A facility storing permanent records must be kept under positive pressure.
- The fire detection and protection system must be designed or reviewed by a licensed fire protection engineer.

- All walls separating records storage areas from each other and from storage areas within the building must be at least three hour fire barrier walls.

- The fire resistive rating of the roof must be a minimum of 30 minutes.

- Automatic roof vents for routine ventilation purposes must not be designed into new records storage facilities.

- Hazardous materials must not be stored in records storage areas.

- Minimum security requirements:
  Control of facility parking
  Receiving / shipping procedures
  Intrusion detection systems
  Adequate exits from record storage areas
  Security locks on entrances / exits
  Visitor control / screening system
  Emergency power to critical systems
  Conduction of background security checks for
    personnel

Federal Survey

The federal survey process is comparable to the state health inspection procedure. The same forms and guidelines are utilized from the Center of Medicare and Medicaid Services with both entities. CMS mandates that random amounts of nursing homes (five percent) are to be inspected at a federal level per year in the nation. Federal surveys concentrate on federal regulatory requirements and do not impose deficiencies for state regulatory statutes. Two major types of federal inspections exist in the United States; observational surveys and look-back surveys.

In federal observational surveys, the federal surveyors are in a facility at the exact same time of state health inspection surveyors; observing and monitoring state surveyors to ensure they are performing state processes correctly, following regulatory guidelines. Look-back federal inspection processes consist of federal surveyors conducting their survey after state surveyors have exited a long-term care facility. This process allows federal surveyors to examine whether their results are consistent with the state health inspection surveyor team processes. When federal and state surveyors are working from the same perception there should be similar deficiencies and scopes of deficiencies cited within a facility in the long-term care industry.

When federal surveys are conducted that generate substandard deficiencies within a long-term care facility; the federal surveyors must notify the state agency of their findings within a reasonable time frame. It is then the State agencies responsibility to notify the Ombudsman, state board licensing the administrator, and all clients' physicians residing in the facility of obtained survey results concerning the nursing home.

Federal surveyors will conduct inspections in facilities that demonstrate no deficiencies during state survey processes more frequently than other facilities. The federal process is utilized to assess if state surveyors and life safety code specialists are performing their jobs effectively and appropriately, as demonstrated in the following scenario.

1. The State Fire Marshall conducted a Life Safety Code Inspection within a facility.

He spent approximately two hours in the facility and cited two deficiencies.

2. Two months later two Federal Surveyors showed up in the same facility to conduct their Life Safety Code survey.

The Federal surveyors spent eight hours in the building and cited thirteen deficiencies.

Quality Indicator Survey

The Center for Medicare and Medicaid Services is in the process of converting the Traditional Survey Health Inspection to the Quality Indicator Survey throughout the United States. A few states have been randomly picked to initiate the new survey process whilch will be rolled out in all fifty states in the future. In July of 2011, twenty-two states and the District of Columbia had been trained in the new survey process.

The new survey process development was initiated in 1993 at the University of Colorado, with a pilot test in 1994 conducted by surveyors in Colorado and Massachusetts. After Senate hearings, CMS then allowed a contract under the leadership of the Universities of Colorado and Wisconsin expand the two-stage survey process to more regulatory regions. Surveyors were trained in the QIS process in September of 2005 in Connecticut, Kansas, and Ohio. In February of 2006, California and Louisiana participated in surveyor QIS training, and Florida participated in October of 2006, and the QIS was implemented in all trained states within the United States. In 2012, Hawaii, Oklahoma, Tennessee, Arkansas, New Jersey, and South Carolina were trained in the new Quality Indicator Survey process.

Stage One consists of preliminary investigations being conducted through resident, family, and staff interviews; client observations; and clinical record reviews. Facility reviews are also performed including: infection control practices, kitchen and dining observations, medication administration, billing processes, quality assurance programs, and analysis of the minimum data set instrument; including both census and admission samples for the evaluation process. Termination of stage one results in Quality of Care Indicators (QCI'S) being formulated that are utilized to identify care areas that require further investigation while progressing into stage two with the survey process.

Stage Two of the Quality Indicator Survey consists of in-depth investigations using Critical Element Pathways that address care planning, care provision, and reassessment. Computerized pathways are mapped to specific "F" tags guiding surveyors in the citing of deficiency processes generated from entered nursing home computerized data. For each unmet critical element the QIS process will display possible "F" tags in the computerized format; surveyors will then implement scope and severity of each "F" tag identified and utilized in the survey processes. Demonstrated below, after the two-stage survey process, are the Critical Element Pathways utilized in the Quality Indicator Survey processes.

QUALITY INDICATOR SURVEY

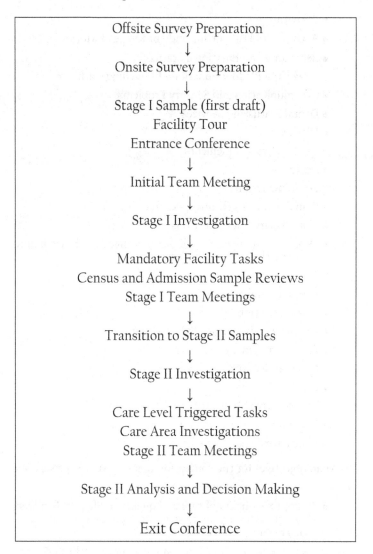

Offsite Survey Preparation
↓
Onsite Survey Preparation
↓
Stage I Sample (first draft)
Facility Tour
Entrance Conference
↓
Initial Team Meeting
↓
Stage I Investigation
↓
Mandatory Facility Tasks
Census and Admission Sample Reviews
Stage I Team Meetings
↓
Transition to Stage II Samples
↓
Stage II Investigation
↓
Care Level Triggered Tasks
Care Area Investigations
Stage II Team Meetings
↓
Stage II Analysis and Decision Making
↓
Exit Conference

The Quality Indicator Survey is a computerized assisted inspection with a two-stage strategy. Survey processes with the new procedure will transpire as follows:

Critical Element Pathways

- Activities
- Activities of Daily Living and / or Range of Motion
- Behavioral and Emotional Status
- Bowel and Bladder Function / Indwelling Catheter
- Communication and Sensory Problems
- Dental Status and Services
- Dialysis
- General Critical Elements:
- Accidents
- Fecal Impaction
- Skin Conditions (bruises, skin tears etc...)
- Non-urinary tract Infections
- Other potential issues (diabetes, congestive heart failure, obstructive pulmonary disease)
- Non-pressure related wounds
- Hospice / Palliative
- Hospitalization / Death
- Nutrition / Hydration/ Tube feeding
- Pain Management
- Physical Restraints
- Pressure Ulcers
- Psychoactive Medications
- Rehabilitation / Community / Discharge
- Ventilator Dependent Clients

Main objectives for the conversion to a new survey process nationwide consists of the following—

- To improve quality of care and quality of life problem identification through more structured consistency and accuracy of survey processes.
- To improve feedback on survey process through time management.
- To provide tools for continuous quality improvement.
- To maintain triggered regulatory areas systematically reviewed and objectively investigated within survey resources.

- To provide enhanced documentation through organizing survey findings with automation.

- To improve survey resources to focus on facilities with the largest number of quality indicator concerns.

It is believed one of the strengths of this survey process is the procedure of utilizing a larger sample group to evaluate systems in nursing home structure will yield more accurate deficiency results. The larger sample consists of up to forty clients residing in a facility at the time of the survey process and up to thirty clients that were admitted within six months of an actual performed QIS survey. The new survey process is more comprehensive than the traditional survey process; resulting in more objective, consistent, focused, and accurate survey findings in long-term care facilities within the nation.

OSHA Survey

Congress generated OSHA (Occupational Safety and Health Administration) from the 1970 Occupational Safety and Health Act formulated in the United States. The organization is responsible for ensuring safe and healthful working conditions for men and women by setting and enforcing standards through providing training, outreach, education and assistance to employers and employees in the nation. OSHA is a part of the Department of Labor covering employers and their employees through federal OSHA or state OSHA programs implemented in the United States.

OSHA will conduct survey processes unannounced and also if requested by a facility to sustain compliance with their regulatory guidelines. OSHA evaluates safety dynamics within employment environments that include —

Blood borne pathogens	*Respiratory protection*
Personal protection equipment	*Exit routes*
Hazard communication	*First aid kits*
Occupational noise exposure	*Fire prevention plans*
Hazardous waste operations	*Infection control*
Lock-out Tag-out	*Emergency responses*
Emergency action plans	*Needle handling & disposal systems*
MSDS – hazardous materials	*Employee TB skin tests*

OSHA surveyors will tour a facility, interview employees, and provide recommendations for deficiencies observed and identified in long-term care nursing institutions. Citations are issued by OSHA surveyors when areas identified are considered unsafe in a facility, with fines of up to 100,000 dollars instituted for unsafe employment environments within nursing home structure.

In 2002, OSHA announced that they would begin inspecting 1,000 facilities out of 2,500 that reported high injury and illness rates under the National Emphasis Program that identified areas of concern within the long-term care industry. Ergonomic back injuries, blood borne pathogens, slips, trips and falls are the focus of the inspections due to accounting for the majority of nursing home staff injuries and illnesses in the United States.

JCAHO Accreditation

The Joint Commission (TJC), previously identified as JCAHO (Joint Commission on Accreditation of Healthcare Organizations) is a non-profit organization that operates accreditation programs for a fee to subscriber hospitals and other health care institutions. State governments acknowledge TJC accreditation as a condition of licensure and Medicare / Medicaid reimbursement processes. The Joint Commission operates on an every three year accreditation cycle with unannounced survey programs conducted in institutions seeking their accreditation services.

All healthcare organizations seeking accreditation through TJC must: be knowledgeable of the organizations current standards of services which are updated yearly on the internet, examine their facilities current processes, institute policies and procedures applicable to TJC standards, and be prepared to improve areas of non-compliance through the survey processes. Institutions must be in compliance with TJC standards at least four months prior to an initial survey. Healthcare organizations seeking The Joint Commission accreditations will have standards evaluated by surveyors encompassing the following specific regions—

Environment of care	*Infection prevention & control*
Emergency management	*Life safety*
Information management	*Nursing*
Medication management	*Security*

Medical staff	Records of care
Safety utilities	Management
Hazardous materials	Leadership
Human resources	Provision of care, treatment services

The mission of the Joint Commission is —

"To continuously improve health care for the public, in collaboration with other stakeholders, by evaluating health care organizations and inspiring them to excel in providing safe and effective care of the highest quality and value."

Several accreditation programs exist depending on the type of healthcare institution or facility being accredited and TJC provides accreditation programs for the following institutions —

Ambulatory Care	Behavioral Health
Critical Access Hospitals	Home Care
Hospitals	Laboratories
Office-Based Surgery	
Long-term Care / Medicare & Medicaid Certification	

A survey team will vary based on the census of a facility and the type of institution being accredited in the nation. However, the team will consist of a nurse, physician, and / or administrative surveyor; and all hospitals have a life safety code specialist included on the survey team for accreditation through The Joint Commission in the United States.

Focus

Extrinsic quality assurance processes are a very important entity in the long-term care industry. Outside organizations governing quality of services provided for elderly clients in the medical field assists in assuring our loved ones are receiving the best healthcare possible in these institutions. All survey processes: traditional, quality indicator, life safety code, complaint investigations, Federal, OSHA, and TJC assist in the continuous quality improvement processes with nursing home reform; assisting in raising the bar within the gerontological nursing profession. The Centers of Medicare and Medicaid Services setting limits for standards of payment for services rendered in long-term care facilities assists gerontological clients residing in healthcare institutions, through implementation of standards that require corporation and middle management attention within the industry.

The improvement of the Traditional Survey process through implementation of the Quality Indicator Survey will aid state surveyors to more accurately identify areas of concern in healthcare institutions throughout the nation, assisting the gerontological or long-term care client to receive the highest quality of care applicable to their specific situation or case. Enhancing extrinsic processes in the long-term care arena through a more focused and accurate survey outcome will delete potentials for biased outcomes in survey processes within nursing homes in the nation, assisting both clients and corporations.

CHAPTER EIGHT. THE CUSTOMER

Diversity of clients encompassing age, ethnicity, culture, medical diagnosis, stay duration, rehabilitation processes, psychiatric diagnosis, and family system interactions generates unique challenges and opportunities in the long-term care industry for healthcare providers. The customer in nursing home structure is not only the client, but anyone who has contact with facilities, including —

Family members	*Visitors*
Vendors	*Physicians*
Therapists	*Sales representatives*
Pharmacists	*Ministers*
Priests	*Surveyors*

The way customers are treated while having contact with individuals employed by a long-term care facility develops the psychological perception and impression of a nursing home. Reputations of long-term care corporations are also formulated by the way nursing home employees interact with customers within the industry.

Customer Service

Customer service is the manner in which businesses provide their delivery systems of specific professional duties to individuals within society. The long-term care industry is no different than any other business when it comes to processes surrounding the formulation, assessment, implementation, and ongoing evaluation of systems that improve and maintain customer service. These system processes will sustain enhancement of quality of care delivery systems and improvement of customer satisfaction in nursing home environments. Good customer service in long-term care facilities will—

- Improve and / or maintain facility reputations
- Decrease staff turnover
- Increase staff morale
- Increase customer satisfaction

Family members and residents judge the quality of services received by what they feel, visualize, and hear while interacting with employees in a nursing home setting. Reliability and consistency of services delivered are two very important aspects surrounding customer satisfaction in the medical field. A clean, well maintained, safe, odor free nursing home environment speaks volumes for the character of a facility and its employees within the long-term care industry. When employees do not care enough about the environment of a facility they are employed to work in within the industry. How can they care about the individuals they are providing healthcare for in the nursing home setting?

Effective customer service also includes answering call lights in a timely manner within a long-term care facility. When visitors or family members see and hear call lights sounding for extended periods of time, it sends a message to the customer, and not a good one. Anticipating individuals needs and following up to ensure needs are met sends a message that staff do care about the clients welfare in nursing home settings, and will decrease call light utilization in the work environment, enhancing customer satisfaction.

Demeanor of staff in long-term care facilities has a huge impact on how businesses are perceived by the public. Hiring the right employees that are people, service and team oriented is a huge portion of the customer service delivery system package. When employees are individuals that possess personality traits of being emotionally engaged with the customer, while performing care services; it improves customer-employee relationships. Healthy business relationships are the building blocks to any industry. When family members and residents feel they are heard and their needs are met it validates the individual and produces satisfied and happy customers. Emotionally engaged employees will develop a connection to a company, generating increased loyalty, and will be driven to deliver high quality services, producing more satisfying relationship connections within the employment arena. Good manners go a long way in the long-term care industry; stating thank-you, please, and I'm sorry can never be over utilized in nursing home structure. Excellent customer service also includes handling individual's complaints in a positive proactive manner, sustaining minimization of future and ongoing problems concerning a family system within long-term care facilities in the nation.

Systems that will set an organizational mindset based on customer satisfaction include —

- The industry's commitment to customer satisfaction.
- Developing ongoing systems to assess quality of services.
- Services delivered based on individuals needs and expectations.
- Providing education and training that is customer oriented.
- Demonstrating respectful relationship interactions in the work environment.

Senior level management in nursing home structure are an important factor surrounding customer satisfaction within the industry. The way employees are treated within an institution will directly affect their satisfaction with their job. Unhappy employees will produce unhappy customers; disrespectful relationship interactions will trickle downhill in an unhealthy business environment generating poor healthcare delivery systems to the clients and family members. Senior and middle level management staff in nursing home structure need to demonstrate to employees in relationship interactions what they want provided to the customer. Reliability, consistency and respectfulness displayed by senior and middle management staff will enhance customer satisfaction within the long-term care industry. Professionals in senior level management positions that are caring, conscientious, speak and listen effectively will set positive examples for lower level staff; encouraging positive relationship attributes to be utilized towards the clients and family members in a nursing home environment.

When employees in senior and middle management positions behave with disrespectful mannerisms; displaying behaviors such as: playing mind games, yelling, profanity utilization towards co-workers, and making fun of individuals in business relationship interactions. It sets a standard for acceptable norms in a business environment, encouraging lower level staff to behave in an unhealthy manner within the employment environment in nursing homes within the nation.

Nursing Home Clients

The elderly, individuals 65 years of age and older, make up around 13 percent of the population in United States. Statistical data show that there are more women than men residing in nursing home environments. Approximately seventy percent of the nursing home population consists of the female gender and two thirds of all nursing home clients have no living relatives. In the nursing home population, an average percentage of clients based on age factor can be visualized as demonstrated below—

85 or older: 44 percent	age 75–84: 32 percent
age 65–74: 12 percent	age 20–65: 12 percent

Racial statistics and cultural beliefs are factors surrounding percentages of clients within the nursing home population. Hispanic cultural beliefs encompass a psychology of taking care of their elderly family members within their home environment, and low percentages of nursing home clients surrounding this race demonstrate that belief system. In 2008, Hispanics consisted of approximately three percent of the totality of nursing home clients in the United States. African Americans round out at approximately twelve percent of the nursing home population in the nation. Cultural beliefs could also contribute to the data in the 2008 statistics, concerning the African American race. Caucasians are the largest racial group of nursing home clients in the United States encompassing eighty-five percent of gerontological patients within the long-term care industry.

Variances in care levels required for individual clients also play a factor in healthcare service delivery systems. Obviously a client that is total care; dependent with food consumption, mobility, hygiene, dressing / undressing, and is incontinent will require more of staffs time versus a client that is partial care or mostly independent in their requirement for healthcare services. Acuity levels of clients need to be assessed and reassessed on a frequent basis to ensure staffing levels are sufficient to meet all clients' needs within a long-term care facility.

The average length of stay for a nursing home resident is between 2.3 – 2.4 years. The Hispanic culture ranges around 1.8 years spent in a nursing home environment within the nation. Not all elderly individuals spend time in a nursing home during their lifespan. The New England Journal of Medicine reported that only 52 percent of all women and only 33 percent of all men 65 years of age or older will spend time in a long-term care environment. Thirty percent of all individuals admitted to a long-term care facility are from a private or semi-private residence within society. The breakdown of pre-admission living statistics are composed as follows—

Residing alone - 12 %
Residing with family members - 15%
Residing with non-family members - 3%

The process of transfers between medical care/nursing home facilities within the healthcare continuum is demonstrated with elderly clients. Eight percent of all long-term care admissions in 2008 comprised of assisted living clients, and approximately 40 percent encompassed acute care hospital transfers. Predictably, the majority of individuals admitted to a nursing home facility are widowed.

Family Systems

Family systems can be conflicted when faced with the decision of placing a loved one in a nursing home; this generates increased stress and feelings of guilt for the individuals responsible for the decision making process. Motivational factors for family systems determining nursing home placement can include caregiver stress due to the burden of responsibility and the demands of caring for a loved one in a home environment, especially as the level of dependency grows. Plus, negative experiences encountered in the role of providing care in or outside of the caregivers' (family members) home environment may increase the potential for nursing home placement.

Evaluating the family system and its utilization of stress adaptation processes can assist medical professionals with a nursing home placement and transition process. It helps to have an understanding of the family system's self-esteem, communication patterns, and rules that govern the family system in relation to societal and environmental factors. Family systems theory and stress process models are two tools utilized that can assist long-term care management and supervisory staff with family involvement in client care within nursing home structure.

The Stress Process Model was developed in 1991 by Leonard I. Pearlin PhD, Graduate Professor of Sociology, University of Maryland, with some revisions made to this concept in the year 1998.

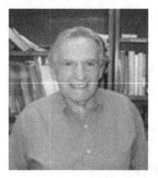

Leonard I. Pearlin, "Stress Process Model"

The Stress Model Theory operates as exhibited in the diagram below —

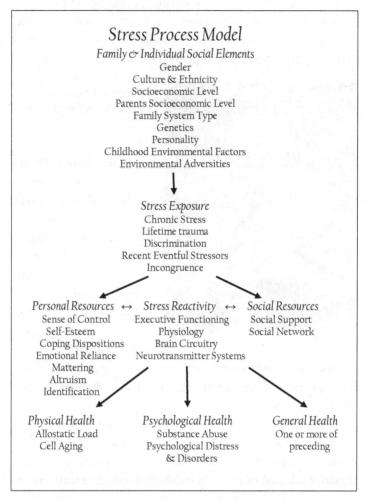

Stress Process Model

Family & Individual Social Elements
Gender
Culture & Ethnicity
Socioeconomic Level
Parents Socioeconomic Level
Family System Type
Genetics
Personality
Childhood Environmental Factors
Environmental Adversities

Stress Exposure
Chronic Stress
Lifetime trauma
Discrimination
Recent Eventful Stressors
Incongruence

Personal Resources ↔ *Stress Reactivity* ↔ *Social Resources*
Sense of Control   Executive Functioning   Social Support
Self-Esteem   Physiology   Social Network
Coping Dispositions   Brain Circuitry
Emotional Reliance   Neurotransmitter Systems
Mattering
Altruism
Identification

Physical Health   *Psychological Health*   *General Health*
Allostatic Load   Substance Abuse   One or more of
Cell Aging   Psychological Distress   preceding
                            & Disorders

The allostatic load is the physiological consequences of chronic exposure to fluctuating or heightened neural or neuroendocrine response that results from repeated or chronic stress exposure in an individual's life. The stress process theory reveals that the way a family system and its members of the system cope with stress; effects outcomes in relationship interactions, physical health, psychological health, social environments, and societal perceptions of the family system.

Family Systems Theory was developed in the 1950s by Dr. Murray Bowen M.D. an American psychiatrist. Dr. Bowen graduated from the University of Tennessee Medical School in 1937 and was a professor in psychiatry at Georgetown University.

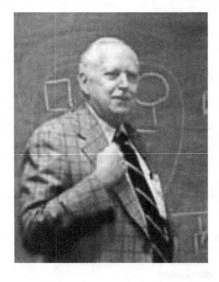

Dr. Murray Bowen, "Bowen Family System Theory"

Family Systems Theory is explained by Dr. Bowen as the family being a unit with individual members and that separate entities cannot be fully understood without examining the family unit as a whole. Family system relationship interaction patterns will effect family units as a whole and individually; providing insight to psychological and physiological dynamics displayed within a family unit. Components of the theory include:

1. There are interrelated elements and structures: Family members and their individual characteristics are the elements that formulate relationships within the family system; including differentiation of self, and variances in individuals regarding their susceptibility to depend on others for their acceptance and approval in the unit. The structure then is the totality of family members (elements) interrelationships including systems and boundaries between the personal and social environment.

2. The elements and structures should interact in predictable patterns. Maintaining equilibrium in the family system and giving individuals the basis on how they will function. Sibling position is a dynamic that effects relationship interactions and patterns within a family unit.

3. All family systems have boundaries whether open or closed. Boundaries are the dynamics that allow individuals to be included or excluded from the unit and maintain a line between the internal / external system. Family systems with open boundaries allow external systems to influence dynamics within the unit. Closed boundaries in family systems isolate its members from external influences and seem self-contained. Emotional cut-off exists with individuals in a family unit when unresolved dynamics occur involving boundaries in a family system to manage perceived problems in the family system.

4. Members of family systems are shaped by rules and messages that are repetitive and redundant within the unit. These dynamics are mostly unspoken, explicit or put in writing; yet exist, inducing power, guilt and control within the family system. Relationship interactions between elements are formulated by these rules and messages evolving in family systems. The family projection process; transmission of emotional, psychological, or behavioral problems from parents to children or children to children will be demonstrated with these unspoken rules and messages.

5. All family systems have subsystems; alliances within the group consisting of 2-3 individuals. Memberships of the subsystems change within the unit and its members have their own rules, boundaries, characteristics etc... Subsystems include triangles; usually two sides in harmony and one in conflict.

Long-term care professionals obtaining understanding of the Stress Process Model and Family Systems Theory will assist in the continuous evolvement of care delivery systems provided to the gerontological client within the long-term care industry. Knowledge base encompassing family system (structure & elements) communication and interaction patterns within a unit can assist healthcare professionals to more fully understand and provide services to the elderly population within the nation through utilizing effective problem solving approaches with family systems in long-term care facilities.

Family centered and elderly friendly environments that address emotional and psychosocial needs of both the client and family members assists in decreasing barriers and maintaining ongoing family relationship interactions in a nursing home setting. Effective communication that allows family members to participate in directing their loved ones care does assist in instilling feelings of safety and security with family members, enhancing satisfaction in psychological perceptions surrounding quality of care services provided for clients in long-term care facilities. Mission statements need to be practiced within a nursing home environment, as they state commitments to addressing needs of the customer. When there is incongruence between the mission and vision of an organization and what is actually practiced within a facility, it sends conflicting messages to the customer; generating stress for both the family and client within the long-term care industry.

Family system adaptation to nursing home placement in a sense can be directly correlated to relationship interactions with nursing home staff and set family system psychological processes that formulate perceptions of those interactions. Health care providers that possess a knowledge base about family system and stress process theories will be better equipped to promote positive psychological outcomes within the nursing home environment for clients and their family units, improving psychological and physical health for customers in the long-term care industry.

Geriatric Care Managers

Geriatric Care Managers are a healthcare specialization focused on gerontology that enables clients to progress through the aging process utilizing community / private based resources and services. Care managers are becoming more popular in the nation. Individuals in geriatric care manager positions may be social workers or nurses with advanced education surrounding geriatric assessment techniques; therapeutic interventions; small business processes; the six domains of care-physical, mental, social, spiritual, financial, and environmental; and care managers must display critical thinking skills. Professional certification as a geriatric care manager is obtained through testing processes with the National Academy of Care Managers in the nation.

Specialists will come into a client's home to perform assessments and develop an operational plan of care generated from the gerontological client's needs at the time of evaluation. Each client assessment will include basic areas of potential concern for healthcare including the following —

Activities of daily living	*Memory*
Safety	*Nutritional status*
Financial circumstances	*Psychological diagnosis*
Medical diagnosis	*Medications*
Family support	*Spiritual needs*
Pain management	

The plan of care developed from the professional assessment is discussed with the client and family members (if needed) to initiate arranging services as required in each particular case. Geriatric care managers will find and implement community resources as needed by a client, assist with facility placement when needed, and provide ongoing educational information to clients and family members assisting gerontological clients through the aging process surrounding met holistic care in the community setting. Diane's case depicts a situation concerning polypharmacy that could be assessed by a care manager in the home environment.

Diane's story

Diane was 86 years old and still living at home with her husband. Due to health status complications over the years, Diane was on several medications to stabilize her chronic disease processes. The situation evolved as follows:

Diane: "George, Do you see those pirates on the neighbor's roof?"

George: "Diane, there are no pirates on the roof."

Diane: "No, George, I am telling you they landed their ship and the pirates are on Pete's roof. Come over here and you can see them for yourself."

George: Complied with Diane's request, then called the physician for an appointment to evaluate his wife.

Diane was experiencing hallucinations, due to adverse chemical reactions from her medications. The medications were adjusted and Diane's symptoms subsided within a couple of days.

Utilizing geriatric care manager service's may assist gerontological clients to stay in their homes for a longer period of time through the process of accurate assessments of client abilities and implementation of interventions to promote well-being for clients in the home environment. Family members may be asked to participate in the client assessment process, especially when memory deficits exist with clients, assisting in enhancing the best possible outcomes for elders in our nation.

Nursing Homes Compare

Nursing Homes Compare is a subdivision of the United States Health and Human Services Department and provides statistical and survey data to individuals about long-term care facilities. The tool contains detailed information about every Medicare and Medicaid certified facility in the nation, allowing individuals to access information surrounding —

Five Star Quality Ratings	*Health Inspection Results*
Nursing Home Staff Data	*Quality Measures*
Fire Inspection Safety	

Health and Human Services generated the five star rating system to provide individuals an availability to compare nursing homes surrounding quality ratings; encompassing the areas of health inspections, staffing, and individual quality measures. A totality is also expressed with one rating for each nursing home institution within the nation.

Quality measures obtained from MDS documentation provide data for determination of star ratings and consist of the number of client cases in a specific nursing home surrounding —

Delirium	*Pain*
Pressure ulcers	*Incontinence*
Mobility decline	*Bedfast clients*
Physical restraints	*Indwelling catheters*
Urinary tract infections	*Weight loss*

Activities of daily living decline
Depression or anxiety increasing
High or low risk pressure ulcer development

There are some limitations with the Nursing Homes Compare process, so it is always a good idea to visit a nursing home facility and contact the State Ombudsman about a prospective client placement to obtain a more accurate assessment process about a specific nursing home in the nation.

The specific areas of evaluation including quality measures do provide criteria for determination and assessment with nursing home placement for the customer. But, further assessment may be required by individuals in some cases; such as a nursing home with a high facility acquired pressure ulcer rate. A nursing home demonstrating this data would need further investigation to determine quality of care provided in the facility. It could be the facility houses many clients surrounding end of life dynamics and pressure ulcer development is inevitable, due to decline in physical statuses from the dying process, or it could be substandard quality of care in the specific nursing home.

Comparisons between nursing homes in the same state will generate a more accurate result; versus two different states. Because, for one, there is currently variation in the health inspection processes between states within the nation. And for two, state licensing nursing home requirements affecting quality of care standards, and Medicaid programs may vary from state to state in the United States.

Staffing data is self-reported once a year by nursing homes and covers only a two week period; thus may not be completely accurate at the time of assessment for customer placement. Quality measures are also self-reported and only contain a few of the areas of care received by clients in the long-term care environment. Potential customers asking direct questions about services delivered in a specific nursing home through staff conversations, or contacting the state Health and Human Services Department can assist individuals with the decision making process regarding family member placement in the long-term care industry within the nation.

Medicare

There are several payment sources for nursing home care coverage and family systems should be knowledgeable about Medicare, Medicaid and Private Pay (nursing home insurance) resources. Medicare is an insurance program developed by the United States government that allows individuals aged 65 or older, people under the age of 65 with certain disabilities, and anyone with end-stage renal disease to obtain benefits for healthcare in the nation. This program also funds residency training rotations for physicians within the United States. A subdivision of the Department of Health and Human Services, (CMS) Centers for Medicare and Medicaid Services administers the processes for Medicare, and the Social Security Administration determines eligibility and processing of payments for this government healthcare insurance program.

The Medicare program is partially funded by payroll taxes that total 2.9% of wages, salaries, and other compensation of employees as imposed by the Federal Insurance Contributions Act and Self Employment Contributions Act developed in 1954. In 2013, the tax will increase to 3.8% for individuals earning over 200,000 dollars a year and joint filling individuals earning over 250,000 dollars per year. It is anticipated by the year 2030, the number of individuals utilizing Medicare benefits will reach 78 million people in the United States. The Medicare program consists of four divisions —

Part A: Hospital Insurance
Part B: Medical Insurance
Part D: Covers Prescription Drugs
Part C: Advantage Plans

Hospital insurance covers all inpatient hospital stays and short term nursing home stays for a specified period. When determining eligibility for long-term care placement the following criteria must be met: a three-day hospital stay preceding admission, the nursing home admission diagnosis and treatment are related to the hospital base stay, and there is a requirement of rehabilitation or skilled nursing services in the long-term care facility. Medicare Part A covers a maximum of 100 days for each specific diagnosis requiring admission; 20 days paid in full and 80 days requiring a co-payment with the insurance program. Co-payment medical insurance can cover some of the services not identified under the Medicare Part A plan coverage.

Medicare Part B typically is utilized on an outpatient basis and goes into effect once a client meets a set deductible and covers 80% of approved services. Some of the services included in this plan are —

Physician services	Nursing services
X-rays	Blood transfusions
Labs	Diagnostics
Renal dialysis	Oxygen
Influenza &pneumococcal vaccines	Chemotherapy
Durable medical equipment	Prosthetic devices

Passage of the Medicare Prescription Drug, Improvement, and Modernization Act in 2006; implemented the Medicare Part D coverage surrounding prescription drug plans. This coverage is not standardized, due to being designed and administered by private health insurance companies that choose which medications, or class of medications that are covered by their specific plan. Medicare does specifically exclude coverage for benzodiazepines, barbiturates and cough suppressants with the insurance coverage.

Medicare Advantage Plans, Part C are designed like an HMO or PPO that are ran by approved private insurance companies. This process works with Medicare paying a fixed rate every month to the insurance provider, and insurance members typically will pay a monthly premium to sustain coverage of items not included in the Medicare A or B plans; such as, dental and vision. Individuals that choose this service will be limited to which primary care providers they can utilize, and will pay out of pocket expenses for utilization of providers not covered by the plan that charge above the allotted amount designated for a provided service.

Within the long-term care industry there are approximately 53,200 Medicare only certified beds, and approximately 609,000 dual certified beds within nursing home facilities in the nation. An average per diem rate of stay is $237.00 per day, and there is an average of 28 Medicare coverage days utilized by most clients in the

United States. Medicare admissions to long-term care facilities accounted for approximately 38% of the totality of admissions in the year 2008 within the nation.

Medicaid

Medicaid is a state managed health care coverage program in the United States that is funded by federal and state governments for individuals and family systems with low income and resources. The fastest growing aspect of this system is the nursing home population. It is believed by the years 2020– 2040 that concerns with state and federal budgets will evolve, due to increased utilization of Medicaid resources within the nation.

In the year 1965, the Social Security Act through Title XIX generated Medicaid services in the United States. The Federal Centers of Medicare and Medicaid Services monitors the program within the states and set standards for eligibility within the nation. In the United States, all states have the option to participate in Medicaid programs, but most states have subcontracted Medicaid services to private insurance companies (Medicaid Managed Care Programs) to provide healthcare coverage to eligible low income individuals within their state.

There are essentially two types of Medicaid, "Community Medicaid" and "Medicaid Nursing Home Coverage. "Community Medicaid assists individuals who have little or no medical insurance in the nation. And, Medicaid nursing home coverage will assist clients with long-term care costs, but individuals are required to utilize their personal income towards the costs of nursing home services; being allowed by the policy to keep $66.00 per month for other expenses. It is estimated that sixty percent of all Medicaid payments utilized assist the elderly population in the United States. Eligibility is not based on poverty alone, other criteria needs to be met and consists of evaluating—

Assets	*Age*
Pregnancy	*Resources*
Disability	*Citizenship*
Blindness	*Lawful immigrant*
Child	

Fraud, unfortunately, has existed in the program with the most abundant amount being more than one million dollars the system was billed by an organized crime group in 2010. The Federal Bureau of Investigation does assist in bringing individuals to justice that tamper with the system that was generated to assist those in need within our nation.

Private Pay

This entity encompasses utilizing personal income and assets to pay for services rendered in the nursing home environment. Personal income can be from several sources including —

Employment pensions	*Social Security*
Interest income	*Dividends*
Bank accounts	*IRAs*
Stocks	*Bonds*
Certificates of deposits	*Real Estate*

Long-term care insurance is also considered to be under the private pay status, it is not a governmental program. Long-term care insurance is formulated to cover the expenses of care in the residence, assisted living, or nursing home environments. Certain health conditions and disabilities are not covered by long-term care insurance policies. Individuals can obtain long-term care insurance privately or through an employer; rates are generally based on age, with monthly payments increasing the older an individual is at the time of purchase of the policy. Policies vary based on daily coverage, overall coverage, deductible, and benefit inflation. In a situation where insurance and other resources do not meet the total payment requirement; clients are required to pay out of pocket for nursing home coverage in long-term care facilities within the nation.

Focus

In the long-term care industry a little over half of the nursing homes are part of a corporate owned chain, approximately 14 % are hospital based, and the remainder are individually owned and operated in the United States. The majority of nursing homes are for profit organizations, with only around 30% being non-profit entities, and seven percent being government owned / managed throughout the nation. Monthly monetary reimbursement in nursing homes averages out at: Medicare eight percent, Medicaid 68 percent, and private pay 23 percent within the long-term care industry. Daily cost rates in nursing homes can range depending on geographic areas, with differences of 91-295 dollars per day charge surrounding care levels in the nation. Alaska and New York range in the higher price rates in the United States. Louisiana and Montana range at the lower price statistics surrounding nursing home care within the nation.

The cost factor encompassing various care levels surrounding nursing home placement is another stress factor for family systems when making decisions about the care of their loved ones within nursing home structure.

Assisting the family system through the process of nursing home placement in the healthcare continuum can be a rewarding aspect of the medical professional's job. Nurses, social workers, geriatric care managers and physicians need to collaborate within the system to provide a smooth transition process from acute care to long-term care, attempting to minimize stress levels for individuals in the healthcare industry. Educating the family system and client through effective communication will assist in minimizing potential adversities within the nursing home environment. Again, healthcare professionals with a working knowledge base about family system function and stress adaptation within the family system; will assist in providing opportunities for growth and development in the nursing home environment for clients and family members in the nation. Hopefully, utilization of this system of processes will assist in sustaining positive outcomes through developed positive psychological perceptions by customers within the long-term care industry and medical profession in the United States.

CHAPTER NINE. ELDER ABUSE

Approximately two million elderly Americans are victims of abuse within the nation annually. It is estimated that for every case that is reported to authorities in the nation, there are between five to ten cases not reported; substantiating a much larger percentage then actually calculated surrounding elder mistreatment in the nation. The majority of elder abuse occurs in the residential environment, but there are some cases that do occur within the long-term care industry. Percentages of gerontological abuse types are approximated as demonstrated below —

Neglect - 60%	Sexual abuse - .04%
Financial exploitation - 12%	Physical abuse - 15%
Emotional abuse - 7%	Other types - .02%

Individuals over eighty years old comprise the largest population involving elder mistreatment. Elder abuse can be described as a single act or repeated behaviors and / or lack of action displayed by individuals that generates harm or distress to elderly human beings in relationship interactions based on trust. It is suggested that ninety percent of incidents concerning elder abuse and neglect are known perpetrators of the victim; such as a spouse, children, or other relatives.

Recognizing Abuse

There are many signs and symptoms that could indicate that an elder is being abused that should warrant further investigation to substantiate or unsubstantiate abuse allegations within the residential or institutional environment. Two indicators are relationship arguments or tension between individuals, and / or changes in personality with an elderly individual. These dynamics identified in relationship interactions could demonstrate signs of potential gerontological abuse. Many other indicators that can be assessed to determine elder mistreatment are demonstrated as follows —

- Physical Abuse: Unexplained bruises, skin tears, hematomas, fractures, sprains, burns, red marks, lacerations, or abrasions. Bodily injury indicative of being restrained. Caregiver refusal for individuals to visualize an elderly client. Providing improper or excessive medications.

- Psychological and Emotional Abuse: Observing belittling, threatening, and/or controlling caregiver behaviors. Emotional liability being demonstrated by an elderly individual; frequent crying, withdrawal, increased confusion, and behaviors that represent dementia-regression. Sleep pattern disturbances. Anxious and fearful behaviors; elderly individual is afraid to make decisions.

- Misappropriation of Property or Finances: Mismanagement of an elders financial resources generating a change in financial circumstances through: stolen money or property; changes in wills, power of attorney, titles and policies; unpaid bills or lack of medical care; and unnecessary services such as, prescriptions, or equipment. Destroying an elder's property.

- Healthcare fraud and abuse: Insufficient staff and training, inadequate responses to questions, duplicate billing or over charging for services, polypharmacy, Medicaid fraud, not providing adequate healthcare, and problematic facilities.

- Sexual Abuse: Physical trauma to genital areas or breasts. Sexually transmitted diseases or unexplained vaginal or anal bleeding.

- Active (intentional) or Passive (unintentional) Neglect: Weight loss, untreated medical or psychological conditions, poor hygiene, dehydration, malnutrition, inappropriate clothing, unsanitary or unsafe living environment, and leaving elderly individuals unsupervised when supervision is required.

- Rights Abuse: Denying civil or constitutional rights of an elderly individual who has not been declared mentally incapacitated.

- Self-Neglect: Not caring for own health and safety. Lack of food or fluids, lack of hygiene, improper clothing for weather, poor shelter, lack of awareness to safety, improper medication utilization, poor environmental cleanliness, and lack of medical attention.

Risk Factors for Elder Abuse

The burden of stress surrounding care giving for elderly clients can be a contributing factor potentially generating mistreatment of elders. Some risk factors to assess with caregivers include the following—

Inability to cope with stress	*Depression*
Lack of support	*Substance abuse*
Caregivers psychological perception (negative)	

Family systems with a history of domestic violence are especially vulnerable to displaying elder abuse within the family dynamics; social history taking can assist in identifying perpetrators at this level. If the elderly client was an abusive individual within relationship interactions during their lifetime, the dynamics they learned could contribute to elder mistreatment in current relationship dynamics. Elderly clients who abuse their caregivers are more prone to counter-abuse in interactions. The following case depicts the potential for this type of situation.

Paul's story

Paul was a 94-year-old, admitted to a long-term care facility due to his declining health. Paul had been married to Lucy his entire adult life and Lucy came to visit him in the nursing home every day. However, Lucy and Paul's marital relationship was abusive and Lucy had been sent home on numerous occasions, because of the abusive behaviors Paul displayed towards her while she was visiting him.

Paul: Yelling loudly at Lucy, "What in the hell is wrong with you? I told you I didn't want a snack, Bitch."

Lucy: "I was just trying to help you."

Paul: Moves off the bed and towards Lucy. Grabs Lucy by the arms and starts shaking her, yelling. "You will do what I say, Do you understand me?"

Staff: Intervenes and sends Lucy home, after talking with her to help her calm down.

Paul: Starts yelling at staff. "What in the hell are you doing? You can't send her home, she is my wife and I can do with her as I please."

Staff: Attempts to explain to Paul that it is not acceptable to yell at his wife or the staff.

Paul: Leans back on his bed, gets a huge grin on his face and states, "Well, well, and just who does this Bitch think she is!"

Staff member: Informs Paul that she will not tolerate his behavior and leaves the room.

Of course, it is not only patients who can be prone to venting frustrations and other negative feelings. Caregivers who lack appropriate training, are delegated too many responsibilities, lack personality traits appropriate for care giving, display a lack of knowledge, have insufficient resources, or work in poor environmental conditions could be prone to displaying elder mistreatment in relationship interactions.

There are some individuals in society who exploit the elderly by developing friendships with isolated gerontological clients. These individuals then take advantage of them, usually financially. Some individuals obtain gratification out of displaying cruelty towards the elderly. An abuser having an ability to demonstrate control and dominance over an elderly human being leads to psychological satisfaction for the abuser in relationship interactions. Individuals who display these behaviors are definitively psychologically ill and should not provide care giving to anyone.

Abuse is related to mental processes; brain neuronal hardwiring gears abusive traits in an individual and abusive human beings utilize abuse tactics to maintain a status of power and superiority over another individual in relationship interactions. Elderly individuals are more susceptible to an abusive personality, due to decline in physical and mental statuses; making them more vulnerable to unhealthy human beings within society. Abusers obtain psychological gratification from their unhealthy behaviors, reinforcing dysfunctional behaviors in relationship interactions. The following graph depicts perpetrator percentages of elder abuse in the nation.

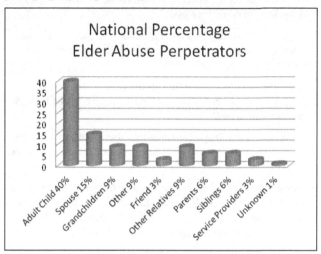

The following case demonstrates how psychological and emotional abuse can occur in the nursing home environment—

Sally's story

Sally was admitted to a nursing home from an acute care hospital due to renal failure, diarrhea, and diabetic ulcers. Sally was a woman that verbalized her thoughts; and this aspect of her personality did not set well with some staff in the long-term care facility.

Some nursing assistants in this particular facility complained to management staff about how much time they had to spend assisting Sally to the restroom, since she was unable to bear her own weight.

Subsequently, Sally was placed on an every-two-hour restroom schedule and was forced to sign a contract stating she would only utilize the restroom every two hours during the day.

Nurse: Entered Sally's room — She was lying in bed crying; she needed to use the restroom and no one would take her, because her two hours had not elapsed.

Sally: "What have I done to get everyone so upset with me? Why does everyone hate me?"

Nurse: Assists Sally into the mechanical lift and to the restroom, ignoring the toileting schedule, due to the patient's diarrhea status.

Sally: Continues crying, while on the toilet, attempting to understand the staff behaviors within the facility. "Why is everyone so mean to me?"

Nurse: Comforts Sally as much as possible, but is unable to explain the cruelty since it was management that instigated the process.

Sally eventually broke out in hives over her entire body due to stress generated by staff cruelty during her nursing home stay, and she was ultimately transported to the community hospital for treatment, never returning to the nursing home facility.

Long-Term Care Prevention and Intervention

Preventative and intervention strategies are mandated to be implemented within nursing home structure by the Federal Government in the nation. Federal guidelines surrounding elder abuse are presented in the CMS manual including: abuse prohibition programs, abuse policies and procedures, and formal education for all staff to be presented on an annual basis. State surveyors will conduct assessments of an abuse prohibition program within each long-term care facility during annual inspection processes and citation of tag F226 is utilized for non-compliance of federal regulatory guidelines. Policies and procedures are required to be in all nursing home institutions that address prevention, identification, investigation, protection, reporting, and facility response of reported investigations.

Preventative interventions that should be implemented in every long-term care facility within the nation include —

Assuring compliance with federal regulations concerning hiring practices through:

- Screening all employees for criminal background checks
- Screening for history of substance abuse or domestic violence
- Screening work ethics
- Screening management abilities of stress and anger
- Screening reactions to abuse

Providing continuing education and training concerning:

- Managing difficult patients
- Conflict resolution skills
- Skills to promote emotional engagement with client
- Stress reduction exercises or techniques
- Witnessing and reporting abuse

Maintaining strict enforcement for reporting of incidents concerning abuse.

Maintaining work environments conducive to healthy relationship interactions through:

- Adequate staffing
- Respect demonstrated by all levels of staff
- Effective communication
- Recognition of employees
- Promoting quality of care

Types of abuse and intervention strategies of elder mistreatment are provided to staff during annual education processes, assisting with the learning curve for all employees in a nursing home facility. Employees are educated annually about processes to follow if they suspect abuse or visualize abuse in the long-term care environment. Suspected abuse requires an employee to report the incident immediately to their supervisor for further investigation by management staff. If abuse is visualized employees are educated to intervene and stop the abuse first, and then report it to their supervisor for management investigation.

There are several entities in the United States to assist individuals suspecting or visualizing abuse of the elderly in our nation including —

- Area Agencies on Aging
- National Center on Elder Abuse (NCEA)
- National Committee for the Prevention of Elder Abuse (NCPEA)
- State Ombudsman
- State Health and Human Services Department
- Adult Protective Services

It is estimated that seventy five percent of all Adult Protective Services reports are related to elder abuse in the United States. Physicians and healthcare professionals encompassed the largest percentage of elder mistreatment reports, with family members being second, and service providers encompassing the lowest percentage of reporters to Adult Protective Services. In most states, it is mandatory by law to report incidents of elder mistreatment. States vary on which individuals in society are required to report suspected abuse, but do include mandatory reporting laws for healthcare personnel, police officers, public officials, social workers, clergy, and counselors.

The following graph demonstrates percentages surrounding individuals in society that report elder mistreatment.

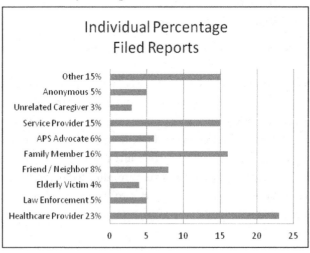

Individual Percentage Filed Reports

Category	Percentage
Other	15%
Anonymous	5%
Unrelated Caregiver	3%
Service Provider	15%
APS Advocate	6%
Family Member	16%
Friend / Neighbor	8%
Elderly Victim	4%
Law Enforcement	5%
Healthcare Provider	23%

National Center on Elder Abuse

The National Center on Elder Abuse (NCEA) was developed in 1988 by the United States Administration on Aging, and was made a permanent resource center in the nation with Title II of the Older Americans Act (1992.) The NCEA utilizes their mission statement as a base for goal setting within the organization and their psychology of their mission is as follows—

> National, State, and local partners in the field will be fully prepared to ensure that older Americans will live with dignity, integrity, independence, and without abuse, neglect, and exploitation.

A mission of prevention of elder mistreatment generates the activity of the organization through educating professionals, educating the public, and providing technical assistance / training to states and organizations in the nation. The NCEA is a resource for policy makers, social service workers, judicial systems, healthcare professionals, elder rights advocates, law enforcement, and researchers. Serving as a major advocate for the elderly, the organization assists in decreasing the number of cases concerning elder mistreatment in our nation. Services provided by the organization include—

- NCEA Website
- NCEA E-News
- NCEA Elder Abuse List Serve
- Clearinghouse on abuse and neglect of the elderly
- NCEA training library for Adult Protective Services and elder abuse

Area Agencies on Aging

State and local Area Agencies on Aging provide a variety of services to elderly individuals within the nation. Services include, but are not limited to: in-home services, center services, transportation, caregiver services, and care management services. Providing these additional services to the elderly population assists them to remain in their residence for a longer period of time, maintaining independence and quality of life.

The National Association of Area Agencies on Aging has a primary mission to build and maintain assistance to elders and individuals with disabilities; encouraging lives lived with dignity and maintaining personal choices for their clients for as long as possible. Departmental services offered by Area Agencies on Aging may include —

Adult Day Care	*Home Repair*
Caregiver Programs	*Case Management*
Employment Services	*Financial Assistance*
Home Health Services	*Home Modification*
Legal Assistance	*Personal Care*
Nutritional Services	*Respite Care*
Senior Housing Services	*Transportation*
Telephone Reassurance	*Senior Center Programs*
Volunteer Services	

Emergency Response Systems
Aging and Disability Resource Center
Elder Abuse Prevention Program
Information and Referral/Assistance Information Services

Adult Protective Services

Adult Protective Services is a component in the Area Agencies on Aging within the nation. All states have programs in place for Adult Protective Services that assist in protecting elderly adults and adults with disabilities that are at risk for mistreatment, neglect, unable to care for themselves, and lack assistance from friends or family members. Case workers from Adult Protective Services programs are generally the first individuals to assess reports of abuse, neglect, and exploitation. Adult Protective Services provides the following systems for individuals in society—

- Receives reports of abuse and mistreatment.
- Investigates alleged complaints.
- Assists law enforcement as required.
- Provides information to county attorneys.
- Assesses adults at risk.
- Obtains court orders for involuntary services.
- Assesses adult's mental capacity for comprehension of circumstances.

- Develops a case plan.
- Initiates service utilization: shelter, medical assistance etc...
- Monitors and evaluates clients and services.

The National Adult Protective Services Association assists in providing education within the United States to professionals in five fields: criminal justice, healthcare, aging services, client services, and financial services. Elder Abuse training requirement assessments are conducted through the National Adult Protective Services association with quarterly training and informational webcasts delivered through this program in the United States.

Ombudsman

The Older Americans Act was amended by congress in 1978 to generate the Long-Term Care Ombudsman program. Systems are established for Ombudsman services in every state and typically are a subsystem within the Area Agencies on Aging.

An Ombudsman is a person who acts as an intermediary between an organization and some internal or external constituent. In the long-term care industry, the Ombudsman acts as an advocate for clients in nursing homes and assisted living facilities. Ombudsman is derived from a Scandinavian word (umbuosmann) meaning representative.

Typically individuals that contact the Long-Term Care Ombudsman are clients, family members, friends, and facility staff; but anyone can contact the department that suspects or visualizes a problem, has a concern or a complaint, and wants to discuss the issue in the industry. Concerns are investigated by the Ombudsman with a psychology of resolving the issue in the client's best interest. Services provided by the Long-term Care Ombudsman are —

> *Education: including residents rights*
> *Information and referral*
> *Consultation*
> *Individual advocacy*
> *Systems advocacy*

Clients' rights in the long-term care industry include, but are not limited to: the right to their own physician, the right to participate in self-medication administration, the right to an individual-ized care plan, the right to voice grievances without retaliation, the right to manage own finances, the right to participate in groups and activities, the right to confidentiality, the right to advance notice of transfer or discharge, the right to protection against unfair eviction, and the right to receive services applicable to individual needs and requirements.

The Long-Term Care Ombudsman is a neutral source located outside of staff and facility structures. An individual in this position has no management decision making power within a facility and practices informally within the nursing home environment. Confi-dentiality is maintained unless a dynamic of serious harm is a po-tential, then Ombudsman personnel may look for someone to make an anonymous phone call to state agencies in this type of situation. An example of an abuse incident that could require Ombudsman utilization occurred in a nursing home setting and was displayed as follows —

A Minneapolis story

In a small town outside of St. Paul, Minneapolis, two teenagers (nursing assistants) engaged in abusive behaviors with clients in the nursing home environment and were legally prosecuted.

The criminal complaint stated that the perpetrators spit in cli-ent's mouths, groped genitals and breasts of some clients, and taunted other clients in the long-term care facility.

One of the perpetrators admitted to getting into bed with a cli-ent and making humping motions, inserting her finger into the client's rectum, and patting the buttocks of other clients while working in the nursing home.

National Committee for the Prevention of Elder Abuse

The National Committee for the Prevention of Elder Abuse was established in 1988 with its main focus centered on understanding abuse and implementing strategies to prevent maltreatment of the elderly in our nation. This organization is one of the three subdi-visions of the National Center on Elder Abuse (NCEA.) Another subdivision of the NCEA is the National Adult Protective Services Association (NAPSA); this organization assists in generating a focus of decreasing elder mistreatment in the United States.

The following graph displays national statistics of elder abuse types in the nation.

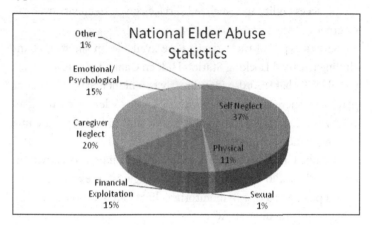

The National Committee for the Prevention of Elder Abuse (NCPEA) is a non-profit organization that provides the following services —

- Conducts research to identify causes for abuse and prevention.
- Identifies critical information needs and participates in exchange of research findings; contributing to the scientific knowledge base on elder abuse.
- Raising awareness of elder abuse.
- Provides education and training to professionals.
- Encourages community coalitions to promote service delivery systems.
- Public advocacy for the elderly in legislative action.

Granny Cams

Granny cams are tiny video surveillance cameras located inside of household items that are utilized to monitor care provided to loved one's or clients inside a residential home or a nursing home. Currently, there is no state that prohibits the utilization of these monitoring devices; Texas and New Mexico are the only states that have legislation that addresses the implementation of a granny cam within a long-term care facility. Some experts perceive that granny cams would assist in building confidence with family members about care provided in the long-term care industry, through providing accessibility to visualized services given to clients over the Internet.

Several types of these devices are available on the market including the iPod Docking Station Hidden Camera that is a tiny internal DVR that records video directly to a hidden SD card for later playback. There are no cables with this type of device, ensuring an ability to utilize the equipment without staff knowledge base in a nursing home environment.

A Cube Clock Radio Hidden Camera that monitors activity in front of the radio at a 92 degree wide angle is an excellent piece of equipment to assist in monitoring client care within the private room only; it requires an AC outlet.

The VersaCam LiveView Desk Clock is a small clock that transmits wireless surveillance to a receiver, connected to a computer (laptop) offering an availability to monitor a client's services provided over the Internet.

The long-term care industry does have some concerns in regards to patient's rights and privacy, especially concerning dressing / undressing and perineal hygiene. Clients that are alert and oriented should be notified by their family members that this type of monitoring is to be utilized, so they can verbalize their thoughts and feelings about being videotaped during private cares, establishing psychological comprehension with a client concerning the utilization of video monitoring devices within the long-term care industry.

Statistics

Nationally, self-neglect is the most investigated report within the nation surrounding elderly mistreatment; caregiver neglect is second and financial exploitation third in demonstrated statistical data. In 2003, there were a total of 565, 800 case reports made to Adult Protective Services concerning adult mistreatment within

the United States; 200, 000 of the reported cases were substantiated nationally. Out of the substantiated reports, the majority of
incidents involved Caucasian females in a residential setting over
80 years old. Every five seconds, an elderly individual is abused in
the nation. In 1996, Adult Protective Services received 293,000 reports of elder mistreatment; with 188, 000 of the reports being substantiated nationally. In the year 2009, there were 55,961,568 cases
reported of elder mistreatment, with 192,243 investigated and fifty
percent of the investigated cases substantiated in the United States.

Instituting educational processes and raising awareness of the
elder abuse problem by national and state entities has appeared to
assist in identifying and addressing dynamics of abuse concerning
the elderly in our nation. Statistical data in this chapter has identified that elder abuse not only exists within the nation, but the number of cases identified substantiates that it is a larger problem then
what most individuals believe to exist within the United States.

The graph below depicts the percentages of substantiated versus unsubstantiated abuse incidents surrounding this dynamic
within a specific state in the nation.

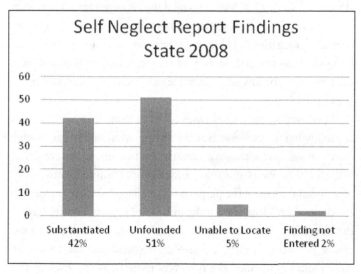

The following case demonstrates a condition of neglect in the
nursing home environment.

Jane's story

The nursing assistants were working the afternoon shift putting clients to bed for the evening in the long-term care facility. Jane was placed on the toilet by a medication aide at approximately 9:00 PM. Shift change occurred at 10:00 PM and the assistants made rounds, but did not check on every resident. Jane was one of the clients not checked.

Jane was found sitting on the toilet at 5:00 AM by the registered nurse on duty. Jane was a stroke patient who could not speak and was paralyzed on the side where the call light was located in the bathroom.

Jane sustained no permanent physical injuries from the incident, so no abuse was substantiated by state surveyors when the incident was reported and investigated. But, how much psychological and emotional trauma did she sustain from the incident?

Specific state reports made to Health and Human Services concluded self-neglect or denial of essential services to be the most common reported and substantiated allegation surrounding elder mistreatment in the nation. In the year 2008, within one specific state there were 2,790 incidents of abuse reported to Adult Protective Services. There is a statistical range of zero to thirty-two percent of all allegations of elder mistreatment substantiated nationally. Neglect has the highest percentage rating and cruel punishment demonstrates the lowest percentage range within data collection in the United States.

When reporting alleged cases to Adult Protective Services have the following information available: name, address, and age of adult victim; name and address of caregiver; nature and extent of abuse; evidence of previous abuse; any other information to identify cause of abuse and identify the perpetrator of alleged abusive incident or incidents. Confidentiality of the individual reporting suspected elder abuse is maintained concerning information provided to a victim or perpetrator, but local law enforcement and the county attorney can be provided the reporters name to assist investigation processes surrounding elder mistreatment. The following graph demonstrates cases identified within two states in the nation.

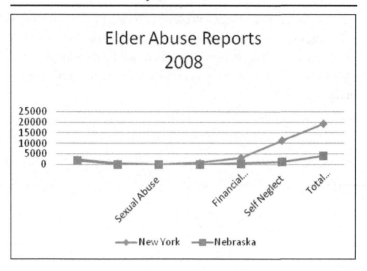

Focus

Unfortunately, abuse of the elderly does occur in our nation and as citizens we need to be observant to signs and symptoms of potential elder mistreatment to assist in decreasing the problem within the nation. Again, the majority of elder abuse occurs in the residential environment and the largest numbers of reported complaints are self-neglect. Services like the National Center on Elder Abuse are wonderful resources to obtain education in regards to this subject matter and assist in identifying, researching, and prohibiting abuse of gerontological clients within the United States.

The long-term care industry does implement its own interventions for prevention and identification as mandated by federal regulatory guidelines, assisting in decreasing the number of cases within nursing home environments. The few cases mentioned within this chapter are the only cases knowledge has been obtained about encompassing a 28 year time span in the long-term care industry within specific states.

Services provided outside of a facility environment like the Long Term Care Ombudsman Program assists individuals that feel their rights have been violated within the industry; assisting to monitor the industry from an outside perspective. Hopefully, with a collaborative effort, nationally we will continue to decrease the number of occurring incidents surrounding abuse of elderly individuals within the country; assisting in providing a healthier lifestyle for gerontological clients, through encouraging processes of aging with dignity in the United States.

Chapter Ten. Rehabilitation Processes

Rehabilitation consists of interventions that physically restore an individual fully or partially that has been injured or disabled from injury, illness, or disease to a functional level supporting quality of life through therapy services. Services provided surrounding rehabilitation processes in the long-term care industry includes restorative nursing, physical therapy, occupational therapy and speech therapy programs.

The perception of long-term care is gradually shifting, due to the number of short stay clients being admitted to facilities within the industry for rehabilitation purposes, and then discharged enabling them to return to their personal residence. Nursing homes or long-term care facilities are expanding from the general perception that it is just an environment for individuals in society to enter just to proceed through the dying process in life.

Therapy programs in nursing homes improve the client's quality of life through restoring decreased capabilities due to trauma, or maintaining current functional levels (preventing decline) through restorative services in the medical profession.

Restorative Nursing

Restorative nursing is a program in the long-term care industry that focuses on maintaining and/or improving a client's functional level. System models utilized for restorative nursing programs differ from facility to facility. Some restorative programs train a few CNAs to be RNAs (restorative nursing assistants); while in other facilities models are implemented with all the nursing assistants being cross trained to be RNAs. Restorative nursing is a nursing function that does not require a physician's order or therapy oversight with service implementation in a nursing home setting. Although, in a lot of cases, restorative nursing is initiated after formalized therapy sessions have finalized; and a therapist or therapists assist in generating a plan of restorative care for the client in a long-term care facility. Other clients are placed on restorative nursing programs when requirements arise such as: pressure ulcers, falls, weight loss, decline in activities of daily living etc.... Services included in a typical restorative nursing program are —

Activities of Daily Living	*Bed Mobility*
Brace / Splint	*Communication*
Ostomy Care	*Locomotion*
Incontinence	*Transfers*
Ambulation / Falls	*Dressing / Grooming*
Range of Motion	*Amputation / Prosthesis*
Eating / Swallowing	
Medication Self-Administration	

Maintenance in a restorative nursing program requires clients to participate in services, and sustain or retain their level of functioning ability with continued program sessions. A client's individual problem or problems must be clearly identified in the plan of care, with goals and interventions stated clearly for each specific client that are measurable and obtainable, qualifying as being realistic for the client in the nursing home environment.

All restorative nursing programs must have a restorative nurse that oversees the program and monitors all restorative assistants during therapy sessions. Restorative nurses formulate and implement client plan of care strategies; while restorative assistants perform specific services and document on daily flow sheets the services rendered to each specific client in the program. The procedure or technique performed for each client must encompass at least fifteen minutes in a twenty-four hour period of restorative nursing to qualify for one day of services. Restorative Nursing programs also vary on how many days' services are provided within long-term care facilities. Some facilities provide restorative nursing seven days a week and over two shifts (days and evenings), while others provide a five day a week program within the nursing home structure.

When reimbursement is sought through Medicare for restorative nursing services, clients must participate in at least two programs during a six to seven day period. Documentation is essential with restorative nursing sessions, weekly charting is not mandatory, but it does assist with monetary reimbursement processes. Weekly chart entries should be performed by a restorative nurse documenting the progression of clients with the plan of care and any sessions that were refused or withheld during the week. Monthly summaries should address the client's progression towards specific goals and their response to treatment. The monthly summary entry by the restorative nurse should also include a synopsis of the client's functional level at the beginning and end of the month, provide explanations of any problems, address modifications to the plan of care, explain goal changes, and identify complications with restorative services rendered in the nursing home.

A quarterly review and chart entry should be made with each MDS completion by the restorative nurse, and included in the review should be the registered nurses assessment of services provided in the long-term care facility. The quarterly review entry should focus on established interventions and if they are meeting each client's goals during restorative sessions. Documentation must also encompass the client's status, abilities, and progression with current treatment modalities or lack of progression with the current plan of care. Nurses must review and modify the plan of care for each client as needed, if client goals are unrealistic, they are deleted and new goals are incorporated to obtain realistic strategies with clients in the restorative nursing program within nursing home structure.

Formal Rehabilitation Therapy

Rehabilitation therapy is a treatment or treatments in the nursing home industry that seeks to restore clients to their previous functional capacity (physical, sensory or mental); increase functional independence; and/or prevent decline of a client's functional status during their long-term care stay. The majority of clients that are on Medicare Part A in long-term care structure receive formal therapy services; due to functional decline from a medical diagnosis of injury, illness or disease. Clients can receive services from one entity such as physical therapy or may be provided services from all three entities physical, occupational, and speech therapy; depending on each specific clients individualized needs within the nursing home environment. Rehabilitation professionals will address a client's physical, psychological and environmental requirements to function in life; improving quality of life through restoring the client's capabilities or modifying physical and social environments to assist the nursing home client through functional capabilities. Rehabilitation therapy services require a physician's order to be implemented with a client in any setting within the medical profession.

Formal rehabilitation therapy includes physical therapy, occupational therapy, and speech therapy. Long-term care facilities vary on how they implement their delivery systems of therapy services. Some institutions hire their own therapists that remain in-house for eight hour shifts; other institutions contract their therapists and they are only available for specific time frames within a day or week in a facility. Physical, occupational, and speech therapists enlist assistance in some long-term care environments due to caseload requirements, and will utilize therapy aides or therapy assistants to ensure services delivered meet regulatory guidelines within the nursing home setting.

Therapists train the therapy aides and aides will perform some of the rehabilitative services rendered in a therapy program within long-term care structure. Therapy aides will assist with tasks of keeping the rehab environment clean, transporting clients to and from sessions, and performing clerical work within the rehab environment in a nursing home. Rehabilitation or therapy aides are trained on the job by therapists, and must possess a high school diploma prior to initiation of on the job educational processes. No state licensing is required to work as a therapy aide in the nursing home environment within the United States.

Rehabilitation or therapist assistants are required to possess an associate's degree from an accredited school for therapy assistants in the nation to work in rehab programs. The American Physical Therapy Association's Commission on Accreditation accredits therapy assistant programs. Therapy assistant programs entail a curriculum that consists of academic and clinical courses to meet therapist's needs for assistance in the industry. Most states require therapy assistants to pass the National Physical Therapy Exam for licensure to practice in their specific state. Under the supervision of a licensed therapist, a therapy assistant will perform therapeutic exercises, electrical stimulation, balance and gait training, ultrasound, massage, compresses, functional equipment utilization training etc... Therapy assistants are responsible for documenting and reporting to the therapist's outcomes from treatment processes with clients under their care in any medical environment.

Some specific diagnosis in the nursing home setting that require formal therapy services are —

Amputations	*Arthritis*
Cardiac Disease	*Stroke*
Neurological Disease	*Fractures*
Spinal Cord Injuries	*Cerebral Palsy*
Traumatic Brain Injuries	*Sprains and Strains*
Pulmonary Disease	*Multiple Sclerosis*

Medicare B services are also provided in the industry with rehabilitation processes. Identification of clients for Medicare B is performed with routine screening interventions during admission and readmission procedures, care plan meetings, quarterly MDS reviews, and any change of client condition. There are many areas covered by the Medicare B plan including —

Restorative Dining	*Dysphagia*
Fall Prevention	*Diet Modifications*
Adaptive Equipment	*Weight Loss*

Environmental Safety	*Range of Motion*
Positioning	*Cognitive Dysfunction*
Functional Nursing Program	
Restorative Nursing Program	

Rehabilitation therapy has demonstrated a challenge of generating evidence that therapy interventions are effective for clients in the gerontological profession and nursing home structure. Formulation of evidence based data through the collection of statistics will assist in formulating a thought process that rehabilitation therapy in the gerontological setting does indeed contribute to function, health and general well-being for customers in nursing home environments. Therapists utilizing strategies for statistical data collection in the industry does assist with generating evidence based principles that addresses subjects and methods surrounding reliability, validity, and client responsiveness to therapy sessions that are evaluated through assessing gerontological methodology practices in the long term care industry.

Outpatient therapy and Medicare part B services are currently being evaluated throughout the nation by a project entitled (DOT-PA) Developing Outpatient Therapy Payment Alternatives. The purpose of the project is to provide data to the Centers for Medicare and Medicaid Services (CMS) on alternate payment methodology. Data collection was obtained during the first six months of 2011 with two assessment tools CARE-C and CARE-F utilized to identify characteristics and therapy outcomes for outpatient services, and the evaluation of data collected through the assessment tools will initiate in the year 2012. Statistical data collected during the project is believed to potentially instigate an impact surrounding Occupational Therapy Services programs provided in medical environments within the nation.

Physical Therapy

Physical therapy is a healthcare profession that focuses on assessment, identification, and implementation of services to maximize quality of life through movement capabilities for a client in the areas of intervention, prevention, treatment, rehabilitation, and promotion. A holistic approach is utilized in physical therapy that addresses physical, emotional, psychological and social criteria for clients; improving their quality of life. Physical therapy assists in restoring the utilization of muscular systems, skeletal systems, and the nervous systems through interventions such as —

- Therapeutic exercises: Range of Motion (active-passive)
- Heat: wax therapy, compresses, baths, short-wave radiation, ultrasound
- Cold: ice packs, cold water soaking
- Whirlpools
- Functional training
- Electrotherapeutic modalities
- Equipment
- Assistive / Adaptive Devices

Physical therapy requires interaction between therapists and clients, but it could also incorporate family members, healthcare professionals and other caregivers with treatment processes within the healthcare industry.

Physical Therapist

A physical therapist in the healthcare profession assesses clients and institutes a plan of care through treatments that reduce pain, restore functional ability, promotes movement, and decreases further functional loss. Physical therapists are trained by accredited physical therapy programs within the nation. The Commission on Accreditation of Physical Therapy Education (CAPTE) accredits entry level academic programs encompassing physical therapy in the United States. All physical therapists are required to maintain licensure in the state of practice after passing the National Physical Therapy Examination with completion of an accredited physical therapy program. Typical accredited educational programs include the following subjects in their physical therapy curriculum—

Biology	*Anatomy and Physiology*
Cellular Histology	*Exercise Physiology*
Neuroscience	*Biomechanics*

Pharmacology	*Pathology*
Radiology / Imaging	*Clinical Reasoning*
Evidence Based Practice	*Diagnostic Processes*
Medical Screening	*Outcome Assessment*
Therapeutic Interventions	

Physical therapists will utilize history and physicals; labs; diagnostic assessments (X-rays, imaging studies); and the medical diagnosis to assist them in developing specific plans of care for clients in the nursing home setting. The time frame of a physical therapy program will vary based on the type of debilitation clients encountered and the client's response to therapy sessions provided. Physical therapists will assess a client's progress, obtainment of specific individualized goals and contact physicians for discharge orders when clients have reached their highest level of functional ability in the rehab environment within long-term care structure.

Occupational Therapy

The World Federation of Occupational Therapists describes occupational therapy as a profession concerned with promoting health and well-being through occupation. Primary goals of occupational therapy are to provide services that establish a client's ability to participate in activities of daily living, promoting quality of life. Activities encompassing an occupational therapy program could be daily living functions, work-related, community based, or extracurricular activities. Occupational therapy may require assistance of family members, friends, healthcare professionals and aides to accomplish plan of care goals surrounding established programs in a nursing home environment. Occupational therapy requires a physician's order to receive services in the long-term care industry.

Occupational therapy may also encompass evaluating social, political and religious factors that inhibit a client's ability to function independently in life. Barriers to effective occupational functioning could also be —

Psychosocial	*Environmental*
Psychological	*Physical*
Cultural	

Occupation in and of itself is an activity in which one engages; and occupational therapy is therapy by means of activity to promote recovery or rehabilitation of clients in the medical profession and nursing home environment.

Occupational Therapist

Occupational therapists work to assist clients with improving and sustaining functional abilities in activities of daily living and work related environments. A major goal of therapist's is to have clients functioning as independently as possible, even with a permanent disability; through modifying tasks or the physical environment. Occupational therapists may require clients to learn new skills; enhancing adaptation to permanent physical or environmental changes in their lives. Implementation encompassing utilization of equipment such as prosthetics and orthotics are an example of this particular approach in occupational therapy. Many activities and interventions encompass occupational therapy such as —

Dressing / Undressing	Food Consumption
Cooking	Therapeutic Exercises
Activities to improve Visual Acuity	Equipment Training
Memory Recall Exercises	Hand-Eye Coordination Exercises
Problem Solving Activities	Abstract Reasoning Exercises
Modifying Work Environments	Modifying Room Environments
Modifying Home Environments	Planning Work related Activities

Again, duration of treatment will depend on services rendered for each specific case and the client's response to treatment strategies implemented in the treatment process. Occupational therapists require a license to practice in their field. Licensure can be obtained by completing an accredited Occupational Therapy Program and passing the national certification exam. Academic programs are accredited by the Accreditation Council for Occupational Therapy Education (ACOTE) in the United States. Occupational therapy training includes theory and skills, physical sciences, biological sciences and behavioral sciences in the curriculum. All accredited schools are required to provide 24 weeks of supervised clinical experience within the program schedule in the nation.

Speech Therapy

Speech therapy is utilized to assist clients to restore speech or correct speech disorders. A client's problems with speech, language or swallowing difficulties generally require some type of therapy intervention. Therapy service interventions are utilized in group, home, or individual settings. Speech therapy is initiated when —

- Speech sounds cannot be produced
- Speech sounds cannot be produced clearly
- Speech rhythm problems are present
- Speech fluency problems are present
- Voice disorders exist
- Swallowing difficulties are evident
- Cognitive communication impairment exists
- Problems are evident with understanding & producing language

Duration of speech therapy interventions is based on each client's disability and response to treatment. Some common diagnoses that require speech therapy implementation are: developmental delays or disorders, brain injury, brain deterioration, learning disabilities, cleft palate, voice pathology, hearing loss, mental retardation, neuromuscular disease, and injury or trauma. Speech therapy requires a physician's order to initiate treatment processes in the medical profession.

Speech Pathologist

Speech therapist or speech language pathologist's work with clients in nursing home settings to improve functional capabilities encompassing individualized interventions through care plan formulation from assessment strategies to improve their quality of life. Some states require their speech therapists to be a graduate of an accredited speech-language pathology program and all speech pathologists must obtain licensure to practice in their specific state. An entity of the American Speech Language Hearing Association called the Council on Academic Accreditation accredits programs for speech pathology training. Passing the National Examination on

Speech-Language Pathology after completion of a Master's Degree program will qualify individuals for practice in the field of speech therapy within the medical profession. Education in a speech pathology program curriculum includes the following—

Anatomy   *Physiology*
Nature of Disorders   *Principles of Acoustics*
Psychological Aspects of Communication
Language and Swallowing Disorders
Evaluation and Treatment of Speech

Communication patterns may have to be tailored to each specific client with implementation of strategies such as sign language, communication boards, picture cards, or the written language as alternative forms of communication. Therapists will also assist clients to strengthen muscles, improve their voices, make sounds, swallow without choking, and deter the possibility of inhaling food or liquid while consuming meals. Family members, healthcare providers and healthcare professionals may be involved in a client's treatment processes to facilitate compliance or increase performance capabilities. In the long-term care industry, speech pathologists are utilized when weight loss dynamics evolve that surround swallowing compensations for clients in nursing homes.

RUG IV Levels

Health Insurance Prospective Payment System (HIPPS) are developed rate codes that display specific sets of patient characteristics that payment reimbursement systems are formulated from in the long-term care industry. The Centers for Medicare and Medicaid Services developed the rate code system for long-term care facilities; Health Insurance Prospective Payment Systems (HIPPS) codes are an alpha-numeric code consisting of five digits. The RUG (Resource Utilization Group) IV level codes are represented in the first three levels of HIPPS codes. Determinations of the levels of specific payment codes are based off data entered on the Minimum Data Set (MDS) assessment tool in the long-term care industry.

RUG levels are also based on therapy services provided and data entered on the MDS (minimum data set) to classify and qualify for Medicare reimbursement with therapy services in the nursing home environment. Therapy minutes and activity of daily living scores (ADL) are two entities that gear some classification of RUG level weight. RUG levels will determine the reimbursement a facility receives for specific clients on Medicare. There are sixteen classifications in this system including —

> Ultra High Rehab Plus Extensive Services: 720 minutes / ADL score 2 or more.
>
> Very High Rehab Plus Extensive Services: 500 minutes / ADL score 2 or more.
>
> High Rehab Plus Extensive Services: 325 minutes / ADL score 2 or more.
>
> Medium Rehab Plus Extensive Services: 150 minute / ADL score 2 or more.
>
> Low Rehab Plus Extensive Services: 45 minutes / ADL score 2 or more.

All the above require tracheotomy care, ventilator / respirator, or isolation for active infectious diseases. Code Examples – RUX, RLX, RUL, RVL, RVX, & RLX.

> Ultra High Rehab: 720 minutes
>
> Very High Rehab: 500 minute
>
> High Rehab: 325 minutes
>
> Medium Rehab: 150 minutes
>
> Low Rehab: 45 minutes and Restorative Nursing

Code Examples – RUA, RVC, RHB, RMB, RLB, RHA.

> Extensive Services
>
> Special Care High
>
> Special Care Low
>
> Clinically Complex

Code Examples – SE3, HE2, LE2, LB1, CC2, CA1, HB1.

> Behavioral Symptoms and Cognitive Performance

Code Examples – BB2, BA1, BA2.

> Reduced Physical Function; Restorative Nursing Services

Code Examples – PE2, PD1, PC2, PB1, PA2.

Resident Assessment Instrument Process

The Resident Assessment Instrument Process in long-term care is mandated by the federal government and consists of the MDS (minimum data set) and CAAS (Care Assessment Areas.) These processes are interventions encompassing clinical assessments of all residents residing in Medicare and Medicaid certified long-term care facilities within the nation; assisting to evaluate functional capabilities and identifying potential problems with clients in nursing home environments.

The minimum data set is completed in nursing homes for two reason bases; Federal OBRA regulations and Medicare Part A PPS schedules. The time frames and reason base are as follows —

Federal OBRA:
Admission (by day 14)
Significant change of status
Not OBRA Required
Significant correction to comprehensive assessment
Significant correction to quarterly assessment
Quarterly
Annual

PPS Assessment:

5-day	*14-day*
30-day	*60-day*
90-day	*Readmission/ Return*
Start of Therapy	*End of Therapy*

The MDS Coordinator completes and submits the MDS forms electronically to the state MDS database; where the data is processed into the National MDS database (Centers for Medicare and Medicaid Services).

In regards to therapy services provided, the MDS has sections specifically for therapists or restorative nurses to complete, or they should provide their data to the MDS Coordinator to be inputted onto the forms; which assists in formulating RUG levels and payment systems for Medicare and Medicaid clients under their care. These areas include the following on the MDS form—

Section O: Therapies:

Occupational Therapy	*Physical Therapy*
Respiratory Therapy	*Psychological Therapy*
Recreational Therapy	

Speech – Language Pathology and Audiology Services

Section O: Restorative Nursing Programs:

Range of Motion (active)	*Range of Motion (passive)*
Splint or Brace Assistance	*Bed mobility*
Transfer	*Walking*
Dressing and / or Grooming	*Communication*
Eating and / or Swallowing	
Amputation / Prosthesis	

Care Assessment Areas (CAAS) are tools that assist in identifying problems for each individualized client, which ultimately will generate care plan formulation specifically tailored to a client's professional requirements in the nursing home environment. CAAS identify specific areas of assessment and include —

Nursing CAAS:

Delirium	*Visual Function*
Cognitive loss (dementia)	*Communication*
ADL/Functional Rehab	*Dental Care*
Incontinence Urinary	*Falls / Restorative*
Feeding Tubes	*Physical Restraints*
Pressure Ulcers	*Psychotropic Medications*
Dehydration / Fluid Maintenance	

Social Services CAAS: ### Activities CAAS:

Psychosocial Well-being	*Activities*
Mood	*Behavior*

Dietary CAAS:

Nutrition
Feeding Tubes

The new MDS 3.0 implemented in 2011, provides for an improved assessment process by incorporating structured interviews throughout the form. Structured interviews increase client participation in collecting and processing of data for assessment duration periods in the areas of cognition, activity, personal preferences, and pain. In section Q the client participates in goal setting, which assists with formulating reality based interventions for clients in the nursing home industry.

Focus

Rehabilitation services are a positive entity in the long-term care industry. Restorative nursing programs assist in maintaining functional abilities for clients, improving their quality of life. Therapy programs enable individuals to regain functional capabilities and return to personal residential environments, or sustain quality of life through functional abilities in the nursing home setting. Proof of positive outcomes with rehabilitation services can be substantiated through data collection within the nation; assisting in continuing positive proactive interventions through rehabilitative processes in nursing homes, maintaining healthcare environments that provide quality of care for elderly clients within the long-term care industry in the United States.

CHAPTER ELEVEN. DEATH AND DYING

Death is defined as the termination of biological functions that sustain a living organism. The word death itself originates from the Old English word "deao." In the United States, legal death is determined by a Statement of Death or Death certificate completed by a licensed medical practitioner. Personhood is legally removed when brain activity has ceased or the ability to resume brain activity is diminished; sustaining legal brain death or biological death. Clinical death or physiological death, "the absence of vital signs" is not by itself necessarily considered a legal basis for pronouncing and individual legally deceased in the nation. Biological death, cessation of brain activity occurs approximately four to six minutes after clinical death.

In 1980, the National Conference of Commissions on uniform state laws formulated the Uniform Determination of Death Act which states: "An individual who has sustained either (1) irreversible cessation of all circulatory and respiratory functions or (2) irreversible cessation of all functions as the entire brain, including the brain stem dead. A determination of death must be made in accordance with accepted medical standards." This legal definition of death was approved by the American Medical Association in 1980 and the American Bar Association in 1981 within the nation.

Dying Process

The dying process is as individualized as the birthing process in life. Each human being will progress through stages in their own way and time frame; some human beings will progress slowly and comfortably, others may progress quickly and uncomfortably. Most human beings will psychologically comprehend their own mortality during the process of dying.

The human body progresses through changes during the dying process; metabolism slows down, decreasing an individual's requirements for food; inducing a decreased appetite and weight loss. Individuals engaged in the dying process may isolate themselves and spend time reflecting on their life. As an individual progresses through stages of death, psychological changes may occur such as disorientation, hallucinations, and delusions. One to two weeks prior to death occurring, an individual usually increases their sleeping patterns; sleeping the majority of time during the day. Physiological changes in the human body initiate as a dying process continues including the following —

- Body temperature decreases
- Blood pressure lowers
- Pulse becomes irregular (slower or faster)
- Perspiration increases
- Breathing patterns change; faster and rapid, then slower or fast and periods of no breathing (Cheyne-Stokes)
- Mottling occurs: purple reddish blotchy discoloration of skin (pooling of blood in extremities)
- Lips and nail beds may become cyanotic (bluish discoloration, due to decreased oxygen to the cells)

Time frames surrounding last stages of the dying process will vary from person to person and can last from days to hours; depending on each individual's psychological and physiological characteristics. Some individuals are uncomfortable during this stage of the dying process and experience pain. Analgesics and narcotics can be prescribed to decrease pain and assist individuals through the dying process in as comfortable of means as possible. Other physiological symptoms may occur such as fluid buildup in the lungs producing congestion; respirations will sound rattled if this occurs. Oxygen may be utilized to assist with labored respirations and suctioning may be performed to remove the secretions. Hearing is the last sense to diminish during the dying process and family members should converse with their love one; providing calming and loving communication.

Religious affiliations (priests or ministers) can be present; providing spiritual comfort for clients and family members during the process of dying. Clinical death occurs when —

- There is irreversible cessation of breathing
- There is irreversible absence of a pulse
- Pallor Mortis occurs (paleness 15-20 minutes after death)
- Livor Mortis occurs (settling of blood lower extremities)
- Algor Mortis occurs (reduction of body temperature)

Family members should always be given an opportunity and be encouraged to stay with the deceased to provide ample time to say their goodbyes; allowing them the time they require for processes of closure. Psychological closure will assist family members during their grieving process of loss in their life. Allowing family members to make decisions such as when the mortuary should be contacted to come to the facility will assist them in their healing process surrounding the loss of a loved one in their lives. The following nurse customer experience about a gentleman being assisted with his dying process will elicit comprehension of educational materials presented.

George's story

George was admitted to the long-term care facility from a local hospital with a nasogastric tube in place and continuous feedings via the tube.

On the day of admission, George was mottled from his toes to his knees, was non- responsive, and kept his eyes closed the entire admission process.

George's wife Mary came every day to sit by his side and talk to him. She would reminisce about their life together, their children, how much she loved him and encouraged him to proceed however he felt he needed to in life, crying at times.

After a week of watching the couple's interactions and George's physiological condition — with mottling increasing up to his waist and his respiration becoming more erratic — the nurse talked with George's wife about the feeding tube, and asked her if she would like it removed. The wife said, "Yes." George's physician was contacted and the nasogastric tube was removed after orders were received from the attending physician.

George died 10 minutes after the tube was removed. As he was dying, his wife sat by his side stating, "I love you. I will always love you." George opened his eyes and looked at his wife the first time since admission and stated, "I love you too."

This experience does indeed demonstrate that the dying individual can hear and comprehend what is being verbalized to them during communication interactions, while the individual is experiencing the dying process during their life.

Stages of Grief

There is variance in belief systems on how many stages individual's progress through during the grief process that range from four to twelve different steps depending on which theory is examined. It is believed by some theorists that the stages are not finitely individualized, yet overlap each other; creating an interaction pattern of back and forth until the grieving individual finalizes their psychological and emotional process. This appears to be more logical, due to grieving steps not being concrete; allowing for the process of differences of characteristics with human beings and their psychology. Grief stages are experienced by dying clients, family members, and can also apply to staff in the nursing home environment that experience loss through the death of customers they have developed emotional attachments to while caring for them in the medical profession.

The different models all appear to be somewhat similar in steps, for the purpose of this discussion we will examine two theories in particular a seven step and a five step stage process of grieving. The seven stages of grief are presented as follows —

1. Shock and Denial - Numbed disbelief can occur with psychological denial of the loss transpiring to protect a human beings emotional and psychological processes.

2. Pain and Guilt - Emotional pain will replace the shock; individuals need to feel and progress through the pain experienced in their life. Some individuals feel guilty thinking they should have done more to help their friend, loved one, or family member.

3. Anger and Bargaining - Emotional feelings of anger are a normal process with grief; some individuals take the anger out on others during this stage. Trying to make deals with God or being angry with God are also typical behaviors that can be displayed during this time period.

4. Depression and Reflection - During this stage individual's typically isolate themselves reflecting on the past. Realization of the finality of loss occurs during the depression and reflection step process.

5. Upward Turn - Emotional, psychological and physical symptomology begins to decrease and adjustment to the loss begins.

6. Reconstruction and Working Through - Restructuring of life begins as an individual initiates returning to a functional capacity in family and social settings.

7. Acceptance and Hope - Emotional pain decreases and individuals psychologically handle the reality of their situation; regardless of what kind of loss has transpired.

The theory encompassing five stages of grief was formulated by Elisabeth Kubler-Ross in 1969 through her book, "On Death and Dying." Dr. Kubler-Ross's proposed stages of grief are —

1. Denial
2 Anger
3. Bargaining
4. Depression
5. Acceptance

Five stage theoretical grief processes contain all the elements displayed in a seven step process model, thus stages are a generalized acceptable belief by theorists concerning the process of bereavement. Individuals will progress through these stages at their own pace and sequencing to obtain acceptance, generating the capacity to move forward with their life. Regardless of which theory is examined the stages buffer an individual's psychological processes; protecting them until they are psychologically able to deal with the finite reality of loss in their life; regardless of what type of loss has transpired for the grieving human being.

Grief Process

It is believed that grief elicits stress, producing pro-inflammatory cytokines and this correlates with activation of the orbitofrontal cortex in the human brain of an individual progressing through grieving processes.

The orbitofrontal cortex is located in the frontal lobe region of the brain; it is involved with cognitive processing concerning decision making and also functions with emotional responses. Grief causes stress linked to emotional processing in parts of the frontal lobe. Grieving processes are inevitable with any perceived loss for a human being; emotional and psychological cycles need to transpire through the grief process for positive healthy outcomes to evolve in an individual's life.

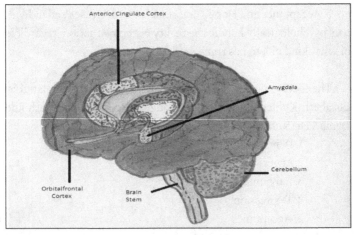

Orbitofrontal Cortex/Anterior Cingulate Cortex/Amygdala

Activation of the anterior cingulate cortex in the human brain also occurs while an individual is grieving. The anterior cingulate cortex is located in the frontal region of the cingulate cortex that forms around the corpus collosum and plays a role in autonomic functions regulating blood pressure, heart rate, and rational cognitive functions such as reward anticipation, decision making, and emotional responses.

Increased activity with the amygdala in the human brain elicits more or deeper sadness during grieving processes. The amygdala is an almond shaped group of nuclei located deep within the media temporal lobes, and has a primary role of processing and memory of emotional reactions.

Long-term care facilities can experience a lot of death and dying dynamics in the institutions, having the perception of God present in individual's psychological processes can be a positive factor in the nursing home environment. Believing in God as a loving entity can assist with psychological aspects of the dying process encompassing gerontological clients and their family members within long-term care structure.

In a new science called neurotheology, it is elaborated on that the belief in God as a loving entity stimulates the anterior cingulate in the brain producing kinder and more compassionate human beings. Gerontological clients deserve to be cared for by kind compassionate human beings before, during, and after the dying process. Saying "God Bless" to clients will assist in the healing process or in some cases the dying process with customers in medical institutions within the nation.

Normal emotional processes that can accompany loss include:

Sadness   *Anger*
Frustration *Guilt*
Shock

The following diagram illustrates the electro-emotionalgram of grief cycles experienced with loss.

High

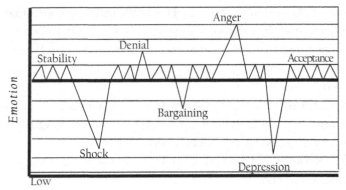

Duration: Days, Months, Years

Physical symptomology with grieving can include fatigue, weakness, shortness of breath, heaviness or tightness in chest region, and dry mouth. An individual's behaviors may alter from normal, such as; demonstrating patterns of decreased food consumption, insomnia, isolation, crying, avoiding reminders of loss, and bad dreams or nightmares may occur while a human being experiences grief in their life. Spiritual disconnect can also transpire during grief processes; especially if an individual is angry with God. Psychological phenomena may be experienced by an individual such as hallucinations, absent mindedness, or preoccupation. The following case depicts the diversity of dying clients in nursing homes.

Ben's story

Two weeks prior to nursing home admission Ben had been living his life, going to work and taking care of his family. Ben was being treated by his physician for thrombosis in his legs when the clots turned to emboli and traveled to both sides of his brain. The medical emergency left Ben brain dead, his EEG showed no activity. Ben was 50 years old and was admitted to the long-term care facility for his last days alive.

Family and friends gathered in Ben's room every day until the day of his death. His wife never left his side from the day of the medical emergency until the morning he passed. The love and caring exhibited by this family and their friends was amazing to watch, and the strength Ben's wife exhibited during her time of very obvious emotional pain left staff speechless.

The family's sense of God was so ever present in this room and place. The family was so appreciative of any little thing done for them and their beloved Ben. During a time of extreme sadness and trauma for the family, they displayed love towards everyone in the nursing home environment.

Elisabeth Kubler–Ross

Elisabeth Kubler-Ross was a Switzerland psychiatrist who railed against what she recognized as mistreatment of terminally ill patients in the 1960s. She spent time studying individuals during the dying process and that led to writing her 1969 book, "On Death and Dying." The five-stage grieving process theory generated by Dr. Kubler-Ross was based on the data she collected from dying patients during her analytical studies.

She graduated from the University of Zurich Medical School in 1957, and relocated to the United States in 1958 to study in New York. In 1962, Dr. Kubler-Ross relocated to the University of Colorado School of Medicine, where she completed her psychiatry training in 1963.

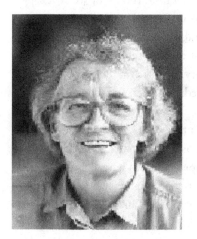

Dr. Elisabeth Kubler-Ross

After completing her psychiatry training, Elisabeth resided in both Chicago and California. Dr. Kubler-Ross died in 2004 at her residence in Arizona. Elisabeth Kubler-Ross was inducted into the National Women's Hall of Fame in 2007. Dr. Kubler-Ross was noted for stating —

In Switzerland I was educated in line with the basic premise: work, work, work. You are only a valuable human being if you work. This is utterly wrong. Half working, half dancing– that is the right mixture. I myself have danced and played too little.

And,

The most beautiful people we have known are those who have known defeat, known suffering, known struggle, known loss and found their way out of the depths.

These persons have an appreciation, a sensitivity, and an understanding of life that fills them with compassion, gentleness, and a deep loving concern.

Beautiful people do not just happen.

Elisabeth Kubler-Ross supported the Hospice movement and denounced euthanasia. Dr. Kubler-Ross felt euthanasia robbed individuals of the right to progress through the necessary emotional and psychological processes of ending their lives.

Hospice Services

Hospice services are a modern day philosophy that encompasses palliative care versus curative care for clients in the medical field. The word hospice originated from the Latin word "hospes" referring both to guests and hosts. Incurably ill clients were permitted into medical practice establishments for the first time in the 11th century, developing the first hospice services delivered during this time frame in medical history. Hospices in the 11th century were a place where the sick, wounded, travelers, and dying could go to obtain rest and comfort.

Modern movement for current hospice service philosophy originated in the 17th century, and was fully formulated in the 1950s by a British registered nurse. Hospice services have not always been viewed from a positive perspective in the medical field, and took several years of development to gain acceptance by all practitioners. Holistic care is practiced with hospice services rendered focusing on physical, emotional, psychological, spiritual, and social needs of dying clients. Hospice practitioners also assist with emotional and psychological needs of family members during and after a client's dying process. Hospice practitioners seek to provide as comfortable of a transition as possible for clients; utilizing medications to alleviate all aspects of pain and discomfort.

Hospice as an established practice in the medical field emerged in the 1980's by opening hospital based programs throughout the nation. In 2008, it is estimated that 1.5 million individuals and their families received hospice services in the United States. Hospice service benefits covered by Medicare also include —

Pharmaceuticals

Medical equipment

Twenty four hour / seven days a week care

Support care for family members after death

Hospice services can be received in hospitals, residential homes, assisted living facilities, veteran facilities, prisons, and long-term care facilities. Hospice practitioners utilize a team approach in care planning with an interdisciplinary philosophy including a physician, social worker, nurse, nursing assistant, volunteers, and a minister or priest. Hospice nurses will provide regular scheduled appointments assessing medical symptoms, pain management, psychological symptoms, and family system needs during a client's dying process. Hospice nurses also keep the physician informed of all assessment processes and findings. A very good book written by two hospice nurses is called, "Final Gifts: Understanding the Special Awareness, Needs, and Communication of the Dying" by Maggie Callanan and Patricia Kelly is a must read for anyone that works with dying patients in the medical field.

Nursing assistants provide daily living requirements such as bathing, food consumption, oral hygiene, and toileting. Social workers assist with emotional and financial aspects concerned with the dying process; setting up systems to aid family members in their community. Ministers and Priests assist with spiritual aspects involved in the dying process for both clients and family members. The multidisciplinary team assists clients and their family members through this inevitable part of life; providing compassionate and emotionally supportive guidance in every aspect of the dying process for those in their care. Hospice services being viewed as a positive aspect in the medical profession assists human beings within society to experience death in as comfortable of a manner as possible; promoting both quality of life and quality of death.

Impact on Staff

In the long-term care industry, death is an inevitable part of the work environment. A facility may encounter several deaths in one month or exhibit sporadic deaths in the institution. Irregardless of the amount of deaths that transpire, end of life dynamics do impact staff within the long-term care industry. In many cases, it involves an individual staff members have taken care of for extended periods of time. Employees in the long-term care industry can experience grief over the death of a client, as any other individual in society. It is not unusual to observe nursing home staff to be crying with family members over the death of their loved one. Healing processes for staff can evolve just as they transpire for family members in the nursing home environment.

The dying process and death is difficult for new certified nursing assistants. A nursing assistant's first encounter with death may be frightful for them in the long-term care environment. Staff needs to be aware of a new employee's feelings in regards to this process of the job requirements and assist them through the task required for post-mortem cares. An experience surrounding an employee's grandpa demonstrates the level of employee-client relationships that can transpire in long-term care environments.

Grandpa's story

Due to a fractured hip, the nurse's grandfather had been admitted to the facility where she was employed.

Grandpa had only been at the facility for about three days when a nursing assistant was rushing him down the hall in his wheelchair from the dining room, and yelling at the nurse to come and assess her grandfather.

Grandpa was placed in bed; he was non-responsive, stethoscope placement over the apex of the heart revealed to the nurse what she had expected. Grandpa had expired. The nurse began crying, holding her grandpa and saying good-bye. The nursing assistants in the room began crying; assisting the nurse with post-mortem cares as they all wept over grandpa's passing.

This experience depicts the level of emotional attachment that exists with some employee-client relationships in the nursing home setting. It is not unusual for employees to have their family members admitted into the facilities where they work, generating a uniquely emotional environment for staff.

Focus

Death is an inevitable part of life. It is something every human being will experience at some time during their transition or journey. Educating ourselves about death; and its physical, spiritual, psychological, and emotional components assists in decreasing fears. A lot of times it is the unknown that generates fear in most individuals; fear of how you're emotionally feeling, fear of how you are physically feeling and fear of the psychological component of the unknown or inexperienced. These components surrounding death can apply to both the dying client and family members in the long-term care industry. Hospice services assist in decreasing these fears for both parties through comforting techniques that include educational processes about the aspects of dying within the experience of life.

CHAPTER TWELVE. ALZHEIMER'S UNITS

Alzheimer's or Special Care Units are those designated regions in a nursing home setting that house clients with dementia diagnosis; assisting in meeting the client's needs and protecting them in long-term care environments. Medical diagnoses that are acceptable for placement on a special care unit include the following —

Alzheimer's Disease	*Vascular Dementia*
Dementia with Lewy Bodies	*Mixed Dementia*
Frontotemporal Dementia	
Creutzfeldt-Jakob Disease	
Wernicke-Korsakoff Syndrome	

Special Care Units are required to conform to specific areas of regulatory statutes that encompass admission criteria, safety, staff training and physical design of a unit within nursing home structure. Clients housed on special care units are at a greater risk for adversities, due to their mental status, and require well trained astute individuals to provide their delivered services within the long-term care industry.

Special Care Unit Regulations

A Special Care Unit shall be a non-institutional home-like environment in nursing home facilities. The physical design of a unit shall assist clients with their activities of daily living and promote all clients safety through —

- A floor plan with limited access to the unit
- A multipurpose room for activities and dining
- Security measures for wandering
- High visual contrasts between walls and floors
- High visual contrast between doorways and walls
- Non-reflective floors, walls and ceilings
- Evenly distributed lighting
- A functional nursing station
- A secured outdoor space and walkways

A unit's floor plan and structure must allow for client freedom of movement in common areas and personal spaces. All corridors and common areas should be free from objects that could potentially generate falls. It is prohibited to lock any client's room on a special care unit in the industry; and locking devices on unit entrance and exit doors shall be electronic releasing when the fire alarm or sprinkler system is activated, or power to the facility fails. Clients should be encouraged to decorate and furnish their rooms as desired in the long-term care environment, and rooms should be identified; assisting clients with recognition of their room on a special care unit. Plus, comfortable rocking / gliding chairs should be furnished in common areas to facilitate calmness with motion movement. A special care unit environment should be free of all toxic plants.

Preadmission screening must be conducted with each potential admission to a special care unit with a substantiating diagnosis of Alzheimer's disease or related dementia obtained during the screening processes. Admission decisions should then be based on a facility's abilities to meet a client's needs, set care levels of a facility, and licensed staff availability on the special care unit within the nursing home.

Due to dementia, behaviors are a common occurrence on a special care unit. Behaviors that are persistent and constitute distress / dysfunction to clients, or present a danger to residents or other individuals in a nursing home are regulated and evaluated as follows —

- Baseline evaluation performed – Concerning intensity, duration, and frequency of behaviors.
- Evaluation of antecedent conduct & activities.
- A client's recent changes or risk factors that could contribute to behaviors.
- Environmental factors that could contribute to a client's actions.
- A client's medical status.
- Effectiveness of behavior management to deter behaviors portrayed in the SCU environment.
- Effectiveness of psychotropic or behavioral modifying medications.

Staffing

There are regulated staffing requirements for a SCU in the long-term care industry. All units first must staff in accordance with rules and regulations governing nursing home facilities, and then special requirements are added to staffing standards to insure quality of services rendered. All SCUs must have a professional social worker or other professional staff member to complete initial social history intakes; develop, coordinate and utilize state or national resources to meet customer requirements; and offer encouragement / support during monthly or bimonthly Alzheimer's support group meetings.

All staff employed to work on a SCU should receive thirty hours of special training within six months of employment encompassing the following topics —

Special Care Unit Policies and Procedures
Etiology, Treatment & Philosophy of Dementia
Effective Communication Skills
Medication Management
Individual Centered Care
Activity Programming
Behavior Management
Alzheimer's Disease
Physical Restraints
Wandering

Ongoing education and training should be provided at least quarterly including the topics of dementia, stages of Alzheimer's disease, behavior problems, behavior management, communication, positive therapeutic interventions, developments and new trends in the industry, and environmental modifications. All educational processes need to be documented for each staff member and kept on file for regulatory review within nursing home facility staff records.

Activities

Activities programming on a Special Care Unit must be directed by a therapeutic recreation specialist, occupational therapist, or an activities professional with two years of experience in programming. The two years of experience with programming must consist of at least one in a full time resident activities program within a healthcare setting. One individual per shift on a SCU will be designated responsibility for activity programming on the unit. Activity programming on a special care unit shall include the following —

Small & large group activities
Social activities daily
Activities geared towards long-term memory
Multiple short time-frame activities
Individual activities
Gross motor activities daily
Self-care activities daily
Sensory & motor activities daily
Outdoor activities weekly (weather permitting)
Sensory & Holiday activities monthly
Crafts weekly
Activities that generate a feeling of usefulness

On a Special Care Unit, client routines shall be structured seven days per week, providing for the possibility of twenty-four hour per day programming, if required. Programming should consist of both planned and spontaneous activities provided to clients on a special care unit. All programs and activities must be appropriate to clients' needs based on cognitive level, beliefs, cultural diversity, values and life experiences.

Programs should also be structured to allow for physical, emotional, and social means of release for clients during activity sessions. Animals, nature and children should be included in programming schedules, as possible, within the special care unit environment. Clients should be encouraged to participate in activity schedules, but not forced to perform any part of an activity the client is not interested in within a nursing home environment.

Reminiscence activities that allow for discussion of past life experiences; incorporating the utilization of photographs, music, special household items etc... could be beneficial for clients in the areas of cognition and mood. Programs that allow for reality orientation and cognitive retraining can assist with improving cognitive capacities, through exercitation of mental abilities, but it has been demonstrated in some clinical trials these types of activities may increase frustration with some clients. An activity director should evaluate benefits versus negative effects of any programming situation and provide services that are best suited for each client's needs. Stimulation programs through recreational activities, pets, children, music, crafts, exercise etc... have demonstrated positive results in the areas of mood and behavior improvement concerning Alzheimer's disease or related dementias in the nursing home environment.

Alzheimer's Disease

Alzheimer's disease is a degenerative, incurable dementia that is associated with plaques and tangles in the human brain. The disease was first diagnosed in 1906 by Alois Alzheimer, a German psychiatrist and neuropathologist. Clinical diagnosis of Alzheimer's disease is obtained through patient history, collateral history from relatives, and clinical observations surrounding behavioral and cognitive testing. Advanced medical imaging can be utilized to rule out other conditions or disease processes assisting with the diagnosis process in the medical profession. A definitive diagnosis of Alzheimer's disease can be obtained through a brain biopsy postmortem. Most individuals who have the disease are diagnosed after 65 years of age, but there are some cases of earlier onset dementia.

There are ten warning signs to observe for possible Alzheimer's disease that include the following—

1. Memory loss that disrupts daily life
2. Challenges in planning, or solving problems
3. Difficulty completing familiar tasks at home, work or leisure
4. Confusion with time or place
5. Trouble understanding visual images or spatial relationships
6. New problems with words in speaking or writing
7. Misplacing things and losing ability to retrace steps
8. Decreased or poor judgment
9. Isolation
10. Changes in mood and personality

Depending on which data is evaluated, Alzheimer's disease can progress through four to seven stages, beginning with the no impairment or pre-dementia stage for all individuals. The second stage (early), in the four-step process, includes stages two (very mild cognitive decline) and three (mild cognitive decline) in the seven-stage model. During these stages diagnosis can be obtained, due to clients displaying noticeable difficulties with obtaining correct word-age, forgetting material read, having difficulties performing tasks, demonstrating problems with planning or organizing, and losing or misplacing objects in their environment.

The seven-step process includes stage four (moderate cognitive decline) and stage five (moderately severe cognitive decline). The Alzheimer's four-step theory labels stage three as moderate. If diagnosis has not been made earlier, it will be made during these stages. Individuals during this time frame will begin to lose the ability to perform normal activities and daily living tasks. Behaviors usually begin being displayed through moodiness, isolating themselves, agitation, wandering, crying and sun downing may start to be exhibited. Cognitive decline continues with confusion increasing; clients will display increased difficulty with recall, simple arithmetic, complex tasks; long-term memory becomes impaired, and delusional symptoms may manifest during this stage.

The last stage is (advanced) in the four-step Alzheimer's theory or stage six (severe cognitive decline) and stage-seven (very severe cognitive decline) in the seven step process. Individuals in these stages will be completely dependent on others for their survival. Progression of the disease process leads to muscle mass deterioration and mobility decline, thus resulting in clients becoming independently immobile. Death usually results from contributing factors of immune and body system decline, resulting in a client's inability to recover from pneumonia or infected pressure ulcers, generated by a client's immobility.

As Alzheimer's disease formulates neurofibrillary tangles and amyloid plaques, it decreases the number of neurons (brain cells) and synapses (connection area between neurons) in the brain. Atrophy then results in the affected regions including the cerebral cortex and subcortical regions, resulting in degeneration of the temporal and parietal lobes of the brain in Alzheimer's patients.

A specific cause of Alzheimer's disease remains to be established, with the most accepted hypothesis being a decrease in synthesis of the neurotransmitter acetylcholine. Acetylcholine is one of many neurotransmitters in the autonomic nervous system and is present in the central and peripheral nervous system. Memory deficits with Alzheimer's disease are associated with a decrease of acetylcholine production in the cholinergic system within the brain.

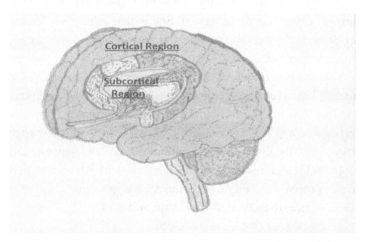

Subcortical and cortical regions

A second hypothesis rests on the belief that amyloid beta deposits in the brain form plaques associated with the cause for Alzheimer's disease. Amyloids are insoluble fibrous protein aggregates that with abnormal accumulation will physically disrupt tissue design and function in the human body.

This theory is based on the chromosome 21 gene and the fact that individuals diagnosed with Trisomy 21 (Down Syndrome) that possess an extra gene copy will exhibit Alzheimer's disease by the age of 40.

Pharmaceutical relief for Alzheimer's disease is currently limited to symptomatic relief. No medication will stop or deter progression of the disease process. There are four medications available on the market—

> Aricept
> Exelon
> Memantine
> Razadyne

Alzheimer's Association

The Alzheimer's Association originated in 1980, and was formulated during a meeting several family support groups attended in 1979 with the National Institute on Aging to discuss the benefits of an organization for Alzheimer's disease within society. Mr. Jerome H. Stone is the founding president of the Alzheimer's Association in the United States.

Today, the Alzheimer's Association consists of a national office and 75 local chapters. It is the largest donor supported organization for Alzheimer's disease in the nation. The Association provides services on a global, national and local level to increase knowledge base about the disease process, offer assistance and support, and improve the quality of care for those inflicted with Alzheimer's disease in the world. Several areas the Alzheimer's Association provides services to individuals in society consists of —

- A 24 hour / 7 day a week helpline.
- Support Groups.
- Educational Programs.

- Alzheimer's Association Green-Field Library.
- Local Chapters.
- Trial Match - Clinical Trials.
- Safety Services: Comfort Zone, Medic Alerts, & Safe Return
- Care Source.
- Walk to End Alzheimer's.

Support Groups

Support groups are a beneficial tool for family members and caregivers dealing with loved ones or clients inflicted with Alzheimer's disease. The disease process can place a great burden on caregivers encompassing physical, psychological, economic, social and emotional components during the duration of the disease. A support group that teaches coping mechanisms in their structure assists with maintaining psychological well-being of at home caregivers, improving home environments for those inflicted with Alzheimer's disease.

There is no specific framework for a support group and variances in structure and style may need to be assessed to establish the correct group placement for an individual's specific needs. Some groups are formal, providing guest speakers and some are informal, allowing for group discussions and verbalizations about the attendee's personal experiences. There are also a percentage of support groups that utilize a combination of formal and informal meetings. Support groups are generally led by medical professionals, social workers or experienced care providers. Three main purposes of Alzheimer's support groups are to —

Teach

Share information

Provide reassurance and encouragement

The environment surrounding support group meetings should be non-judgmental and confidential, allowing individuals to obtain the assistance they require while dealing with the Alzheimer's disease process. Meetings can vary in occurrence: weekly, biweekly, monthly, or bimonthly. There generally is no charge for these meetings and they typically last around two hours for each session. Some support groups have a faith or religious based element. Group sizes will vary; there is usually a limit between six to twenty individuals, providing ample time for all to verbalize and ask questions as desired during the session or meeting. For many individuals, support groups are the one place they feel comfortable and understood when they verbalize their feelings and challenges while dealing with the Alzheimer's disease processes in their life.

Memory Walk

The Alzheimer's Association Memory Walk initiated in 1989, it is the nation's largest event to increase awareness about Alzheimer's disease in the United States. Memory Walks throughout the nation aid in obtaining funding for research, care, and support for those inflicted with the disease in their family systems. Currently, the event is held in over 600 locations nationwide with typical walk regions ranging from one to three miles. Participants are asked to raise funds through tax deductible donations; monetary amounts collected are utilized within the community of an event participation, assisting those inflicted with Alzheimer's disease in a participant's hometown.

Memory Walk affiliates encourage team building for this event through the formation of national, company and family teams. Teams should consist of ten to twelve individuals, and the Association will provide tools to assist individuals interested in team building for the Memory Walk event. The Memory Walk event has assisted with the monetary aspects concerning this disease process raising over 260 million dollars nationally, assisting family members and those inflicted with Alzheimer's disease in the nation. The following case assists in the comprehension within society that when taking care of individuals experiencing psychological dysfunction, in most cases, we need to step into their world to resolve problems.

Raylene's story

Raylene had lived in the nursing home for approximately a year and had been admitted, due to cognitive decline resulting in the inability to care for herself in her personal residence. Dinner was being served in the dining room and Raylene had refused to leave her room to eat.

Nurse: *"Raylene, it's time for lunch. You need to not skip your meals."*

Raylene: *"I can't leave, the children are under my bed and I have to take care of them."*

Nurse: Looks underneath the bed and asks, *"There are children under your bed?"*

Raylene: *"Yes, the children need help."*

Nurse: Gets down on her knees, looks under the bed and starts motioning for the children to come out from under the bed, saying, *"Okay, children, it's time to stop playing hide and seek, we need to go home now."*

The nurse proceeds to walk the children out of the facility, so they can go home. Raylene goes to the dining room for lunch after she follows the nurse and watches the children leave the facility. Psychologically, Raylene was content, believing the imaginary children had come out from under the bed and gone home

Focus

Alzheimer's or Special Care Units are a needed entity in the long-term care industry to provide safety and effective care delivery systems for clients afflicted with dementia within the healthcare continuum. These units must provide activities as directed in federally mandated guidelines; assisting with the quality of life for dementia clients residing in nursing home environments. All special care unit employees should be well trained to address quality of care issues that transpire with the Alzheimer disease process, contributing to an increase of quality care delivery services within the medical profession.

As scientific research continues to uncover the specific causes for Alzheimer's disease, hopefully eliciting treatment modalities to decrease the progression of the disease process or to potentially cure the disease in the future. The long-term care industry will adjust their care delivery services provided to adapt to current trends and standards of practice within the medical profession.

CHAPTER THIRTEEN. OPPORTUNITIES IN THE INDUSTRY

Opportunities for improvement in care delivery systems within the long-term care industry encompasses many different strategies, systems, evaluations, interventions, implementations, and monitoring techniques; including an ability to self-evaluate nursing home facilities in the healthcare continuum. We have discussed several of these systems and / or monitoring tools including survey processes, tracking systems, educational processes, training, and corporate intervention strategies within the gerontological medical profession. Assistance of individuals developing tools such as the Eden Alternative, Family Systems Theory, Stress Process Model, and Quality Indicator Survey processes demonstrates that improvement of care for the gerontological client is a continuous evolvement of entities from all institutions within society. As we progress into the future, there will be many more avenues to assess and monitor surrounding the gerontological nursing profession in long-term care structure.

Types of employees within the nursing home environment do indeed affect the care delivery systems for gerontological clients. Employees that are emotionally engaged with clients and possess a desire to improve systems surrounding healthcare for the elderly in our nation will effectively deliver better quality of care in a nursing home setting. Hiring practices and retention of employees plays a huge factor in the type of services gerontological clients receive in the long-term care industry. Thus, we will begin this discussion by first evaluating staff burn-out, retention, and staff morale within the nursing home industry.

Staff Burn-Out

Employee burn-out, the exhaustion of physical or emotional strength occurs in the long-term care industry, due to levels of care delivery systems required surrounding gerontological clients in nursing home environments. This process generates perceived negative stress by an employee over a prolonged period of time. It is not unusual for one CNA to be responsible for the care of 10-12 clients during their shift and many times nurses are responsible for 60-100 clients during a single rotation. Staff to patient ratios being set at this level does contribute to exhaustion for employees and a decreased quality of care delivery systems within nursing home structure.

Corporate owned nursing home facilities set what is called PPDs (allotted hours per day per patient) ratios that dictate staffing levels within nursing homes. The federal regulation F353 tag states –

> The facility must have sufficient nursing staff to provide nursing and related services to attain or maintain the highest practicable physical, mental, and psychosocial well-being of each resident, as determined by resident assessments and individual plans of care.

To calculate a facilities PPD take the total number of nursing hours scheduled and divided it by the facility or unit census. Example: a facility has 540 nursing hours scheduled and the patient census is 165, the PPD would be 3.27. Once the PPD is calculated for a facility the PPD can then be multiplied by the number of clients, giving the nursing department total scheduled hours for a unit. Example: PPD 3.27 x 105 (census) equals 343.35 nursing hours.

The problem with PPD's is that they are calculated based off of numbers, not care levels of patients in the nursing home environment. So, while a facility may have fewer numbers of clients it could be that their level of care is higher requiring two assist with services delivered or more complicated procedures, such as IV"s or trach's, yet these factors will not be evaluated within PPD composition surrounding nursing hours for a long-term care facility.

Employees most likely to develop burnout are typically the best employees. The employee prone to burnout takes their job seriously; puts more time into their work, and actually cares about their work performance. Stress from the burnout lowers the immune system and burnt-out employees are prone to more illnesses. Allowing employees some individuality, choices, control, creativity and diversity with their job performance will assist in decreasing the possibility of burnout in the work environment. Staff burnout contributes to employee's being less perceptive in their work performance as exhibited in the following case.

Elvin's story

Elvin was admitted to the nursing home after a total hip replacement procedure. His foley catheter had been removed prior to long-term care placement. Incontinence dynamics contributed to an infection process developing in the incision line with subsequent packing and IV Vancomycin ordered.

The staff did not notice an infection process was occurring until the incision line began opening up in areas where it had been healed.

Elvin's incision line rehealed with packing removal and IV antibiotic utilization, but the entire process probably could have been alleviated with more astute staff looking after him.

Staff Morale

"Morale" is the capacity of people to maintain belief in an institution or a goal, or even in oneself or others, and for them to pull together persistently and consistently in pursuit of a common purpose. Psychological and emotional attitudes of staff in regards to tasks within the nursing home environment are a necessity for management to evaluate, assisting in providing continuous quality improvement systems. Factors that can contribute to staff morale positively or negatively include:

Layoffs	*Work Culture*
Cancelling Benefit Programs	*Team composition*
Lack of Union Representation	*Perceived Status of Work*
Cancelling Overtime	*Realistic Opportunities*
Job Security	
Management Style	

Poor employee morale should be addressed as soon as it is identified within an institution or organization, because it will contribute to burnout for employees. Poor employee morale is generally a reaction to other negative events within the work environment and will spread to others on a team through psychological manipulation, thus eventually generating a perpetual cycle of problems if not addressed in a timely manner. Simply asking employees what they perceive as the problem is one easy step to utilize to obtain definitive reasons for negative attitudes and perceptions in the work environment.

Improving employee morale should be a process that is taken seriously within nursing home structure in the nation. Management teams in long-term care facilities need to acknowledge and praise successes in the work environment; individually and as a team. Supervisors also need to be honest, trustworthy and fair in their relationships and interactions, assisting to establish a healthy employment environment. Maintaining effective communication by listening and actually hearing employees will help avoid misunderstandings, improving staff morale and staff retention.

Staff Retention

Maintaining employees in their positions is a major dynamic in the long-term care industry that impacts healthcare delivery systems. Longevity of employees adds to sufficient staffing numbers to provide care to our elderly, and sustains knowledge base encompassing client preferences and desires in their home environment. Employee retention decreases turnover, training costs, and loss of talent in the business setting. Individuals in management positions within the long-term care industry need to evaluate valence within their organizations structure; insuring that the rewards offered by the institution align with the needs employees seek to fulfill in their work environment. Low valence will decrease job satisfaction, increasing turnover, thus decreasing retention of employees in nursing home facilities; which directly affects care level delivery systems.

Maslow's hierarchy of needs has been utilized in some organizational structures to assist in maintaining retention of employees. The five areas in Maslow's hierarchy of needs are: self-actualization, esteem needs, psychological needs, safety needs, and social needs. Organizations meeting employee's self-actualization and esteem needs appear to have increased retention in the work environment in some institutions. The cost factor of utilizing this strategy has not proven to be beneficial in comparison to retention numbers according to some experts, thus it is not utilized in great efforts within most business cultures.

Decreasing turnover in the long-term care industry is an ongoing process in nursing home structure. The following are a few strategies to potentially utilize to assist with the retention dynamics:

- Base interviews on the match of an applicant and the organizations excellence.
- Invest in training.
- Have results based job descriptions.
- Define performance excellence.
- Coach excellence.
- Celebrate the importance of each job.

Staffing Impact on Quality of Care

Staff morale, staff turn-over and staff retention have impacts on the safety and quality of healthcare delivery systems provided for gerontological clients in the long-term care industry. Analytical research in the area of nurse/nursing sensitive outcomes or patient outcomes potentially sensitive to nursing; can be limiting, due to the availability of data regarding quality measures in the healthcare profession. Yet, it is widely accepted that patient care outcomes can be directly correlated to nursing services provided, and the environments in which services are rendered to patients within the medical profession.

The American Nurses Association conducted a study poll in 2008 concerning this topic with the following results obtained:

> 73% of nurses do not believe that staffing is sufficient in their area of practice.
>
> 59.8% left direct care jobs because of insufficient staffing.
>
> 51.7% of nurses believe the quality of nursing care is declining.
>
> 48.2% would not feel confident having a loved one in the area they are currently employed.

Work environments in the long-term care industry are influenced by employee morale, retention, turn-over, burn-out, and agency utilization in the nursing entity. These dynamics can interfere with budgets, continuity of care delivery systems, standards of care, workload for employees, psychological health of clients, and knowledge base of employees providing nursing services within an institution. Several studies of these work environmental factors demonstrate that increased weight loss, increasingly ungroomed residents, lower functional improvement of residents, and higher facility-acquired pressure ulcer rates were directly correlated to care delivery systems, in other words, were outcomes that were related to the quality of nursing care.

Low staffing levels increase the workload for nursing personnel, which increases employee turn-over rates, thus decreasing the knowledge base of personnel within an institution; and both affect the quality of care delivery systems. The Centers for Medicare and Medicaid Services (CMS) utilize and provide the quality care indicators data or quality measures data to other entities within the nation; attempting to make nurse sensitive outcomes visible to society, increasing knowledge base about this dynamic in the medical profession. Sufficient staffing levels ensure quality of care delivery services in the long-term care industry as depicted in the following story.

Sara's story

Sara was a dementia patient that was fairly aggressive with care-givers, requiring restraint utilization to maintain IV placement for medication administration. One afternoon the nursing home staff levels were depleted, due to sick calls and burnout staff unable to assist with overtime. Sara could remove her wrist restraints if not applied adequately and on this particular afternoon, Sara did perform this act.

When the charge nurse walked into the room and saw that the restraints were removed and on the floor, she began assessing the central line site to ensure patency and safety.

Observation by the nurse revealed that the Groshong tube had been torn in half with part of the tube still inside the resident and the other part of the tube on the floor. The nurse applied a hemostat to the torn central line tube still inside the resident to decrease air flow into the tube.

The physician was contacted and subsequently the resident was sent in for surgery to correct the malfunctioned tube. The question that arose in the nurse's mind, though, was, "How long did the resident lie in bed after removing her restraints and damaging the central line prior to staff discovering the incident?"

Other factors that influence quality of care delivery systems include specific nurse characteristics such as knowledge base, experience, fatigue, dedication, mental health, physical health, and / or drug / alcohol utilization. Nurse related serious errors usually lead to complications and poor clinical outcomes for residents in the nursing home setting. The organizational nursing home environment encompassing support systems, climate, culture, management styles, communication systems, and corporate involvement will influence resident outcomes in the long-term care industry. Gerontological clients are initially at a higher risk for obtaining poor outcomes from the quality of care provided to them simply because of their age, sometimes their voices are not heard, and complaints are simply written off as "old age." Family members, in a lot of cases, become very strong advocates for their loved ones in the nursing home environment, and justly so.

The following diagram depicts the dynamics that go into play effecting both quality and quantity of care delivery systems in the long-term care industry.

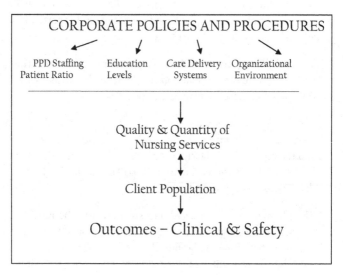

CORPORATE POLICIES AND PROCEDURES

PPD Staffing Patient Ratio   Education Levels   Care Delivery Systems   Organizational Environment

Quality & Quantity of Nursing Services

Client Population

Outcomes – Clinical & Safety

Community Involvement

Several entities of community involvement encompass the long-term care industry, and higher community involvement does demonstrate to promote increased levels of care delivery services within nursing home environments. Individuals in society need to have an increased awareness that their level of participation in nursing home structure does assist in improving care services provided to gerontological clients within the medical healthcare continuum. Through community involvement including religious affiliations, volunteers, support groups, and organizations that educate on gerontology; as a society we can ensure the best possible care delivery services are being provided for our elderly in the United States.

Religious Affiliations

Religious gerontology is the study of religion among older adults and across the lifespan. Organized religious activities appear to increase adjustment to the aging process for many individuals within society. Studies have demonstrated that religious involvement is a psychologically and physically therapeutic factor in the lives of older adults; regardless of gender, social class, race, ethnicity, nationality, study design, or religious affiliation. It is suggested that religious involvement will discourage risk-taking behaviors, provide social supports, instill beliefs that encourage peacefulness, and enhance coping skills surrounding stress; thus decreasing the development of disease processes through various religiosity components.

Religion and the geriatric population can induce scientific studies within the specialty areas of epidemiology, psychiatry, medicine, and sociology. In epidemiology, it appears that pathogenesis will decrease in individuals actively affiliated with religious organizations within their social structure. Medicine, in current decades has begun to accept the linkage between religion and disease, but has been unable to fully incorporate it into the medical practice. Although, medicine and nursing do tend to view a holistic approach to healing including psychological, physical, spiritual, and social components. Psychiatry does not practice at a high level surrounding religious beliefs and health. It is believed by some that Freudian negative beliefs encompassing religion; influences belief systems of the psychiatric community within the nation.

Sociology has become the front runner in research studies surrounding the correlation between religion, health and aging. It is believed that this science will continue to push for empirical evidence supporting a linkage between the entities, improving the quality of life for gerontological clients in society and within nursing home structure.

God is ever present in nursing home environments through the beliefs of clients, family members, staff, clergy, and priests; promoting religiosity in the long-term care industry. The nursing home environment encourages client attendance of religious services to promote psychological and emotional health. Also, death and dying events that are a part of the long-term care environment; often take place in the presence of religious figures, and clergy involvement can provide comfort and assistance to family members after their loss of a loved one within long-term care structure. The study of the correlation between gerontology and religion will be a topic of ongoing interest to individuals within the long-term care industry, encouraging and promoting holistic care of clients within nursing home settings in our nation.

Volunteers

Volunteers are a much needed equity to assist in providing quality of life dynamics encompassing many activities in the long-term care industry. Volunteering is the act of assisting other individuals through work, or assisting a specific cause without monetary reimbursement for services. Activity Directors are the individuals that generally recruit and seek retention of individuals for volunteer programs in the nursing home environment. Most long-term care facilities employ a full time activity director that seeks to enhance life experiences for clients within their home, and accomplish this task with ongoing activities that require volunteers to meet the schedules of life enhancing programs provided. Volunteers engage in generally altruistic activities that benefit others; enhancing client quality of life in nursing home environments within the nation.

The volunteer in the long-term care industry may assist with implementing group activities such as bingo, crafts, card games, or assist with holiday programs and meals. Some individuals will volunteer their skills encompassing singing, instrument playing, and painting demonstrations. One institution had an attorney donate his time to meet with family members to discuss end of life legal processes, assisting the family members of clients in the nursing home through educational processes surrounding death. The scope of what volunteer programs can provide customers in the long-term care industry is wide ranged and can vary based on specific needs in different geographical areas within the nation.

In any case, volunteers in many situations have been forerunners with initiating many different services for the gerontological population within the long-term care industry. It appears that the major dynamic with volunteer programs is maintaining retention of volunteers in the industry. Individuals within the long-term industry and in society need to recognize the importance of volunteers that donate their time to assist the elderly in our nation by implementing volunteer recognition programs and rewarding longevity of volunteering individuals within our nation.

The Long-term Care Ombudsman program is a dedicated group of volunteers who give their time to residents in nursing homes. Ombudsman volunteers will advocate on the residents behalf encouraging them to age with dignity, autonomy and choice. Volunteers for this program give clients a stronger voice through resolving complaints, visiting residents, conducting facility assessments, training facility staff, and investigating complaints in the nursing home environments within the United States.

Support Groups

Support groups encompass a wide range of variance surrounding the specific bases for providing group meetings in the nursing home environment. These groups are generally established to provide assistance through educational materials; relating personal experiences; listening to others; providing sympathy, empathy and compassion; and developing social networks. Some examples of different support groups available in the nation that assist individuals involved with the long-term care industry include:

- Caregiver support groups
- Bereavement support groups
- "Going On" support groups
- Diabetes support groups
- Adult children on aging parents support group
- Caring for caregivers
- Adults caring for loved ones
- Alzheimer's support groups
- Fronto-temporal dementia caregiver support group
- Brain injury & stroke support group
- Lou Gering's disease support group
- Parkinson's support group
- Amputee support group

- Complex/ heavy care support groups

These types of meetings do enhance coping mechanisms for caregivers and family members surrounding the delivery of services, or through general understanding of disease processes; improving the quality of life for family systems in the long-term care industry. Most developed support groups are "open" and allow all individuals that are interested to attend, but there are some cases of limitations set on the numbers of individuals that can participate in each session. In any situation, it is a positive approach to call ahead of time to gain information about each support groups activities, ensuring adherence to their standards.

The following case displays the level of confusion with dementia clients in the nursing home environment that can be experienced at any given moment during their day and how a support group could assist family members with the nursing home placement decision process, surrounding client confusion and emotional responses.

Betty's story

Betty had been a client in the long-term care facility for an extended period of time and her dementia had increased over the years. One evening Betty was extremely upset, crying over the fact she had been placed in the facility by her family without her prior knowledge.

Nurse: "Betty, I know this is hard, but your family was thinking of your best interest. You need to shut you beautiful eyes and attempt to get some sleep. It is two o'clock in the middle of the night and we are not able to handle this problem until morning."

Betty: "My child. Have you completely lost your mind? There is no way I can shut my eyes and go to sleep when I am driving the car."

Focus

There are several areas that require a multidisciplinary approach with improvement of care delivery systems within the long-term care industry. As we progress towards the future, with gerontological populations continuing to increase as longevity develops further in the lifespan, our nursing homes in the nation are required to evaluate and develop interventions to resolve opportunities experienced or exposed in the long-term care industry.

Opportunities should be looked at positively, assisting in enhancement of holistic care approaches for the gerontological client. The few opportunities mentioned in this chapter are a basis for a beginning within the long-term care industry to assist corporations, gerontological clients, nursing home staff, family members, and the medical community to move forward continuing to improve quality of life strategies for the gerontological population in the United States.

ACKNOWLEDGEMENTS

I would like to thank all of the patients and family members who have so patiently and lovingly let me take care of them and their loved ones in nursing homes throughout the United States. It is because of you and for you that this book evolved and was written. I deeply appreciate every one of you and the educational, psychological and emotional gifts that we have experienced together while working towards your goals in the long-term care environment within the medical field.

Delia

RESOURCES

Alzheimer's Association. http://www.alz.org/alzheimers_disease

Eden Alternative. http://wwwedenalt.org

Family Systems Theory. Bowen Theory. http://www.thebowencenter.org

National Center on Elder-Abuse Statistics. http://www.ncea.aoa.gov/ NCEAroot/Main_Site

Nursing Home Statistics. http://www.efmoody.com/longterm/nursingstatistics.html

Strategic Management. Quick MBA. http://www.quickmba.com

Stress Process Model. http://www.jstar.org/discover/10.2307/2/36676?uid

United States Department of Health and Human Services. Federal Centers for Medicare and Medicaid Services. State Operations Manual. 5-23-2011. Publication: 100-07.

Photos:

Dr. Andrew Kramer picture. http://www.nursinghomequality.com

Dr. Leonard I. Pearlin picture. http://www.bsos.umd.edu/socu/people/ faculty/lpea

Dr. William Thomas picture. http://pickerreport.org

Dr. Elisabeth Kubler-Ross picture. http://www.nlm.nih.gov

Dr. Murray Bowen picture. http://ffrnbowentheory.org

INDEX